Biological and Molecular Aspects of Mast Cell and Basophil Differentiation and Function

Biological and Molecular Aspects of Mast Cell and Basophil Differentiation and Function

Editors

Yukihiko Kitamura, M.D.
Departments of Pathology and Internal Medicine
Osaka University Medical School
Osaka, Japan

Shoso Yamamoto, M.D., Ph.D.
Department of Dermatology
Hiroshima University School of Medicine
Hiroshima, Japan

Stephen J. Galli, M.D.
Department of Pathology
Division of Experimental Pathology
Beth Israel Hospital, and
Department of Pathology
Harvard Medical School
Boston, Massachusetts

Malcolm W. Greaves, M.D., Ph.D., F.R.C.P.
St. John's Institute of Dermatology
St. Thomas's Hospital
London, United Kingdom

Raven Press 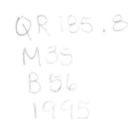 New York

Raven Press Ltd., 1185 Avenue of the Americas, New York, New York 10036

Made in the United States of America

Library of Congress Cataloging-in-Publication Data

Biological and molecular aspects of mast cell and basophil
    differentiation and function / editors, Yukihiko Kitamura . . . [et
    al.]
           p.   cm.
    Includes bibliographical references and index.
    ISBN 0-7817-0314-X
    1. Mast cells—Congresses.   2. Basophils—Congresses.   I. Kitamura,
Yukihiko.
        [DNLM: 1. Mast Cells—immunology—congresses.   2. Mast Cells-
-physiology—congresses.   3. Basophils—immunology—congresses.
4. Basophils—physiology—congresses.   5. Cell Differentiation-
-congresses.   QS 532.5.C7B615 1995]
    QR185.8.M35B56 1995
    616.07'9—dc20
    DNLM/DLC
    for Library of Congress   95-2737

The material contained in this volume was submitted as previously unpublished material, except in the instances in which credit has been given to the source from which some of the illustrative material was derived.

Great care has been taken to maintain the accuracy of the information contained in the volume. However, neither Raven Press nor the editors can be held responsible for errors or for any consequences arising from the use of the information contained herein.

Materials appearing in this book prepared by individuals as part of their official duties as U.S. Government employees are not covered by the above-mentioned copyright.

9 8 7 6 5 4 3 2 1

Contents

I. Cytokines Involved in Mast Cell and Basophil Development and Function

Contributing Authors

Hermine Agis

Department of Internal Medicine I
Division of Hematology
The University of Vienna
Währinger Gürtel 18-20
A-1090 Vienna, Austria

Akikazu Ando

Department of Pediatrics
Kurume University School of Medicine
67-Asahi-machi
Kurume-shi
Fukuoka 830, Japan

Ken-ichi Arai

Department of Molecular and
*   Developmental Biology*
The Institute of Medical Science
The University of Tokyo
Shirokanedai 4-6-1, Minato-ku
Tokyo 108, Japan

Naoko Arai

DNAX Research Institute of Molecular
*   and Cellular Biology*
Department of Cellular Biology
901 California Avenue
Palo Alto, California 94304-1104

Jonathan P. Arm

Department of Medicine
Harvard Medical School, and
*   Department of Rheumatology and*
*   Immunology*
Brigham and Women's Hospital
250 Longwood Avenue
Boston, Massachusetts 02115

K. Frank Austen

Department of Medicine
Harvard Medical School, and
*   Department of Rheumatology and*
*   Immunology*
Brigham and Women's Hospital
250 Longwood Avenue
Boston, Massachusetts 02115

Robert M. Barr

St. John's Institute of Dermatology,
*   UMDS*
St. Thomas's Hospital
Lambeth Palace Road
London, SE1 7EH United Kingdom

Peter J. Bianchine

Allergic Diseases Section
Laboratory of Clinical Investigation
National Institute of Allergy and
*   Infectious Diseases*
National Institutes of Health
NIH Building 10, Room 11C210
Bethesda, Maryland 20892

John Bienenstock

Faculty of Health Sciences
McMaster University
1200 Main Street West, Room 2E1
Hamilton, Ontario L8N 3Z5 Canada

John J. Costa

Departments of Medicine and Pathology
Beth Israel Hospital and Harvard
*   Medical School*
330 Brookline Avenue
Boston, Massachusetts 02215

Vince Duronio

The Biomedical Research Centre and
*   Department of Medicine*
The University of British Columbia
2222 Health Sciences Mall
Vancouver, British Columbia
*   V6T 1Z3 Canada*

Hideharu Endo

DNAX Research Institute of Molecular
*   and Cellular Biology*
Department of Cellular Biology
901 California Avenue
Palo Alto, California 94301-1104

David M. Francis
St. John's Institute of Dermatology,
  UMDS
St. Thomas's Hospital
Lambeth Palace Road
London, SE1 7EH United Kingdom

Hiromi Fukamachi
Division of Immunobiology
La Jolla Institute for Allergy and
  Immunology
11149 North Torrey Pines Road
La Jolla, California 92037

Stephen J. Galli
Department of Pathology
Division of Experimental Pathology
Beth Israel Hospital, and
Department of Pathology
Harvard Medical School
330 Brookline Avenue
Boston, Massachusetts 02215

Arturo Genovese
Division of Clinical Immunology and
  Allergy
University of Naples Federico II
School of Medicine
Via S. Pansini, 5-80131
Naples, Italy

Malcolm W. Greaves
St. John's Institute of Dermatology,
  UMDS
St. Thomas's Hospital
Lambeth Palace Road
London, SE1 7EH United Kingdom

Michihiro Hide
St. John's Institute of Dermatology,
  UMDS
St. Thomas's Hospital
Lambeth Palace Road
London, SE1 7EH United Kingdom

Thomas F. Huff
Department of Microbiology and
  Immunology
Virginia Commonwealth University
1101 East Marshall Street, Box 980678
Richmond, Virginia 23298–0678

John E. Hunt
Department of Medicine
Harvard Medical School
Department of Rheumatology and
  Immunology
Brigham and Women's Hospital
250 Longwood Avenue
Boston, Massachusetts 02115

Akihiko Iemura
First Department of Pathology
Kurume University School of Medicine
67-Asahi-machi
Kurume-shi
Fukuoka 830, Japan

Susumu Itoh
Department of Blood Transfusion
Shinshu University School of Medicine
Matsumoto 390, Japan

Tohru Itoh
Department of Molecular and
  Developmental Biology
The Institute of Medical Science
The University of Tokyo
4–6–1 Shirokanedai, Minato-ku
Tokyo 108, Japan

Tomoko Jippo
Departments of Pathology and Internal
  Medicine II
Osaka University Medical School
Yamada-oka 2–2, Suita
Osaka 565, Japan

Yoshikazu Kameyoshi
Department of Dermatology
Hiroshima University School of
  Medicine
Kasumi 1–2–3, Minami-ku
Hiroshima 724, Japan

Yuzuru Kanakura
Departments of Pathology and Internal
  Medicine II
Osaka University Medical School
Yamada-oka 2–2, Suita
Osaka 565, Japan

Tsutomu Kasugai
*Departments of Pathology and Internal
    Medicine II
Osaka University Medical School
Yamada-oka 2–2, Suita
Osaka 565, Japan*

Toshiaki Kawakami
*Division of Immunology
La Jolla Institute for Allergy and
    Immunology
11149 North Torrey Pines Road
La Jolla, California 92037*

Yuko Kawakami
*Division of Immunobiology
La Jolla Institute for Allergy and
    Immunology
11149 North Torrey Pines Road
La Jolla, California 92037*

Zaisun Kim
*Department of Immunology
Juntendo University
School of Medicine
Hongo 2–1–1, Bunkyo-ku
Tokyo 113, Japan*

Yukihiko Kitamura
*Departments of Pathology and Internal
    Medicine II
Osaka University Medical School
Yamada-oka 2–2, Suita
Osaka 565, Japan*

Chris S. Lantz
*Department of Microbiology and
    Immunology
Medical College of Virginia
Virginia Commonwealth University
Box 678 MCV Station
Richmond, Virginia 23298*

Hyun-Jun Lee
*The Institute of Medical Science
The University of Tokyo
Shirokanedai 4–6–1, Minato-ku
Tokyo 108, Japan*

Julie A. Leftwich
*Department of Microbiology and
    Immunology
Medical College of Virginia
Virginia Commonwealth University
Box 678 MCV Station
Richmond, Virginia 23298*

Kevin B. Leslie
*The Biomedical Research Centre and
    Department of Medicine
The University of British Columbia
2222 Health Sciences Mall
Vancouver, British Columbia
    V6T 1Z3 Canada*

Donald W. MacGlashan, Jr.
*Division of Clinical Immunology
Johns Hopkins Asthma and Allergy
    Center
5501 Hopkins Bayview Circle
Baltimore, Maryland 21224–6801*

Gianni Marone
*Division of Clinical Immunology and
    Allergy
University of Naples Federico II
School of Medicine
Via S. Pansini, 5–80131
Naples, Italy*

Esteban S. Masuda
*DNAX Research Institute of Molecular
    and Cellular Biology
Department of Cellular Biology
901 California Avenue
Palo Alto, California 94304–1104*

Sayako Matsuoka
*Division of Immunobiology
La Jolla Institute for Allergy and
    Immunology
11149 North Torrey Pines Road
La Jolla, California 92037*

Dean D. Metcalfe

Allergic Diseases Section
Laboratory of Clinical Investigation
National Institute of Allergy and
  Infectious Diseases
National Institutes of Health
NIH Building 10
10 Center Drive MSC 1888
Bethesda, Maryland 20892–1888

Hugh R. P. Miller

Department of Veterinary Clinical Studies
The University of Edinburgh
Veterinary Field Station, Easter Bush,
Roslin Midlothian EH25 9RG
Scotland, United Kingdom

Mitsunobu Mio

Department of Pharmacology
Faculty of Pharmaceutical Sciences
Okayama University
Tsushima Naka, 1–1–1
Okayama 700, Japan

Toru Miura

Division of Immunobiology
La Jolla Institute for Allergy and
  Immunology
11149 North Torrey Pines Road
La Jolla, California 92037

Atsushi Miyajima

Department of Cell Biology
DNAX Research Institute of Molecular
  and Cellular Biology
901 California Avenue
Palo Alto, California 94304–1104

Eishin Morita

Department of Dermatology
Hiroshima University School of Medicine
Kasumi 1–2–3, Minami-ku
Hiroshima 724, Japan

Makoto Murakami

Department of Medicine
Harvard Medical School
Department of Rheumatology and
  Immunology
Brigham and Women's Hospital
250 Longwood Avenue
Boston, Massachusetts 02115

Kenji Muraoka

Department of Clinical Oncology
The Institute of Medical Science
The University of Tokyo
Shirokanedai 4–6–1, Minato-ku
Tokyo 108, Japan

Akihiko Muto

Department of Molecular and
  Developmental Biology
The Institute of Medical Science
The University of Tokyo
4–6–1 Shirokanedai, Minato-ku
Tokyo 108, Japan

Yoshiyuki Naito

DNAX Research Institute of Molecular
  and Cellular Biology
Department of Cellular Biology
901 California Avenue
Palo Alto, California 94304–1104

Tatsutoshi Nakahata

Department of Clinical Oncology
The Institute of Medical Science
The University of Tokyo
Shirokanedai 4–6–1, Minato-ku
Tokyo 108, Japan

Koji Nakamura

Department of Dermatology
Hiroshima University School of Medicine
Kasumi 1–2–3, Minami-ku
Hiroshima 724, Japan

George F. Newlands

Moredam Research Institute
Edinburgh, Scotland, United Kingdom

Ko Okumura
Department of Immunology
Juntendo University
School of Medicine
Hongo 2–1–1, Bunkyo-ku
Tokyo 113, Japan

Nobuo Okumura
Division of Clinical Chemistry and
* Medical Technology*
School of Allied Medical Sciences
Shinshu University School of Medicine
Matsumoto 390, Japan

Chisei Ra
Department of Immunology
Juntendo University
School of Medicine
Hongo 2–1–1, Bunkyo-ku
Tokyo 113, Japan

John J. Ryan
Department of Microbiology and
* Immunology*
Medical College of Virginia
Virginia Commonwealth University
Box 678 MCV Station
Richmond, Virginia 23298

Hirohisa Saito
Division of Allergy
National Children's Medical Research
* Center*
Tokyo 154, Japan

Nobukuni Sawai
Department of Pediatrics
Shinshu University School of Medicine
Matsumoto 390, Japan

John W. Schrader
The Biomedical Research Centre and
* Department of Medicine*
The University of British Columbia
2222 Health Sciences Mall
Vancouver, British Columbia
* V6T 1Z3 Canada*

John T. Schroeder
Johns Hopkins Asthma and Allergy Center
5501 Hopkins Bayview Circle
Baltimore, Maryland 21224–6801

Lawrence B. Schwartz
Department of Internal Medicine
Division of Rheumatology, Allergy, and
* Immunology*
Medical College of Virginia
Virginia Commonwealth University
1102 East Clay Street, Box 263
Richmond, Virginia 23298

Cheryl L. Scudamore
Department of Veterinary Clinical Studies
The University of Edinburgh
Veterinary Field Station, Easter Bush
Roslin Midlothian EH25 9RG
Scotland, United Kingdom

Giuseppe Spadaro
Division of Clinical Immunology and
* Allergy*
University of Naples Federico II
School of Medicine
Via S. Pansini, 5–80131
Naples, Italy

Richard L. Stevens
Department of Medicine
Harvard Medical School
Department of Rheumatology and
* Immunology*
Brigham and Women's Hospital
250 Longwood Avenue
Boston, Massachusetts 02115

Mineo Takagi
Department of Pediatrics
Shinshu University School of Medicine
Matsumoto 390, Japan

See-Ying Tam
Departments of Pathology
Beth Israel Hospital and Harvard
* Medical School*
330 Brookline Avenue
Boston, Massachusetts 02215

Ryuhei Tanaka

Department of Clinical Oncology
The Institute of Medical Science
The University of Tokyo
Shirokanedai 4–6–1, Minato-ku
Tokyo 108, Japan

Toshihiko Tanaka

Department of Dermatology
Hiroshima University School of Medicine
Kasumi 1–2–3, Minami-ku
Hiroshima 724, Japan

Kenji Tasaka

Department of Pharmacology
Faculty of Pharmaceutical Sciences
Okayama University
Tsushima Naka 1–1–1
Okayama 700, Japan

Mindy Tsai

Department of Pathology
Beth Israel Hospital and Harvard
  Medical School
330 Brookline Avenue
Boston, Massachusetts 02215

Kohichiro Tsuji

Department of Clinical Oncology
The Institute of Medical Science
The University of Tokyo
Shirokanedai 4–6–1, Minato-ku
Tokyo 108, Japan

Tohru Tsujimura

Departments of Pathology and Internal
  Medicine II
Osaka University Medical School
Yamada-oka 2–2, Suita
Osaka 565, Japan

Risako Tsuruta

The Institute of Medical Science
The University of Tokyo
Shirokanedai 4–6–1, Minato-ku
Tokyo 108, Japan

Peter Valent

Department of Internal Medicine I
AKH Wien
Division of Hematology and
  Hemostaseology
The University of Vienna
Währinger Gürtel 18–20
A-1090 Vienna, Austria

Sumiko Watanabe

Department of Molecular and
  Developmental Biology
The Institute of Medical Science
The University of Tokyo
4–6–1 Shirokanedai, Minato-ku
Tokyo 108, Japan

Melanie J. Welham

The Biomedical Research Centre and
  Department of Medicine
The University of British Columbia
2222 Health Sciences Mall
Vancouver, British Columbia
  V6T 1Z3 Canada

Barry K. Wershil

Departments of Pathology
Beth Israel Hospital and Harvard
  Medical School
330 Brookline Avenue, and
Combined Program in Pediatric
  Gastroenterology
The Children's Hospital and
  Massachusetts General Hospital
Boston, Massachusetts 02215

Hideo Yagita

Department of Immunology
Juntendo University
School of Medicine
Hongo 2–1–1, Bunkyo-ku
Tokyo 113, Japan

Shoso Yamamoto

Department of Dermatology
Hiroshima University School of Medicine
Kasumi 1–2–3, Minami-ku
Hiroshima 724, Japan

Libo Yao

Division of Immunobiology
La Jolla Institute for Allergy and
Immunology
11149 North Torrey Pines Road
La Jolla, California 92037

Masahiko Yasuda

Department of Immunology
Juntendo University
School of Medicine
Hongo 2–1–1, Bunkyo-ku
Tokyo 113, Japan

Takashi Yokota

Department of Molecular and
Developmental Biology
The Institute of Medical Science
The University of Tokyo
Shirokanedai 4–6–1, Minato-ku
Tokyo 108, Japan

Preface

Our understanding of the molecular basis for basophil and mast cell development and function has increased tremendously over the last few years. Mast cells and basophils are important factors in many disorders with components of immediate hypersensitivity, such as atopic dermatitis, allergic rhinitis, and certain forms of anaphylaxis and asthma, as well as in some types of urticaria. However, recent findings have indicated that these cells may participate importantly in a variety of other disorders with inflammatory and/or immunological components, including rheumatoid arthritis, scleroderma, inflammatory bowel disease, and psoriasis. In addition, the recent recognition that mast cells represent a potentially important source of a broad spectrum of multifunctional cytokines has renewed interest in the roles of these cells in such basic biological processes as wound healing, angiogenesis, fibrosis, and cancer. Thus, mast cells and basophils are now regarded as having relevance in biology and medicine that extends far beyond their roles in immediate hypersensitivity.

In many immunological, inflammatory, or pathological processes, the mast cell population at the site of the response can change markedly in size and/or important characteristics of phenotype. Although these phenomena have been recognized for many years, they are only now becoming understood in molecular terms. The recognition that the c-*kit* ligand, stem cell factor, represents a major regulator of the survival, development, and function of mammalian mast cells represents only one of the important milestones in the recent rapid progress in our understanding of the molecular regulation of mast cell development and function. In turn, the mast cell has served as a valuable and versatile model system to investigate the molecular biology of interactions between stem cell factor and its receptor, and to identify and functionally characterize additional tyrosine kinases, and other elements of signal transduction pathways, which can be shared by a wide variety of clinically important cell types.

This book brings together contributions from many of the leading investigators in the biology and molecular biology of mast cells and basophils, and presents a broad but detailed consideration of the current understanding of the development and function of these fascinating cells. This volume should provide valuable new information of special interest to allergists, dermatologists, hematologists, immunologists, rheumatologists, cell and molecular biologists, pharmacologists, and pathologists. We hope it will also help to foster additional efforts to elucidate the molecular basis for basophil and mast cell development and function.

Acknowledgments

This book contains invited papers given at an international symposium entitled "Biological and Molecular Aspects of Mast Cell and Basophil Differentiation and Function" that was held on June 16–18, 1994, in Hiroshima, Japan. We are very grateful to the sponsors listed below, and especially to Sansho-Kai, an organization of dermatologists in Hiroshima, whose generous support significantly contributed to the success of our symposium. The publication of this book was supported by a generous contribution from YASUDA Medical Research Foundation, Osaka and Tokyo, Japan.

Many colleagues helped us to organize the meeting. We thank them for their help, and especially, we thank the moderators of the sessions at the meeting, Ken-ichi Arai, K. Frank Austen, John Bienenstock, Dean D. Metcalfe, John W. Schrader, and Kenji Tasaka, for so ably performing their duties.

We thank the many individuals in the Department of Dermatology, Hiroshima University School of Medicine, who assisted in the local organization of the meeting. They not only helped the meeting to run smoothly but provided the participants with a moving and memorable introduction to the culturally and historically important city of Hiroshima.

Finally, we thank the conference participants. Their eager contributions of information, opinion, and discussion not only represented the basis of the meeting's success but also constituted a fine example of international understanding, cooperation, and good will.

Bayer Yukuhin, Ltd.
Daiichi Pharmaceutical Co., Ltd.
Dainippon Pharmaceutical Co., Ltd.
Eisai Co., Ltd.
Fujisawa Pharmaceutical Co., Ltd.
Hitachi Chemical Co., Ltd.
Kabi Pharmacia Diagnostics K. K.
Kaken Pharmaceutical Co., Ltd.
Kanebo Ltd.
Kissei Pharmaceutical Co., Ltd.
Kowa Co., Ltd.
Kojin-Kai
Kyowa Hakko Kogyo Co., Ltd.
Lederle (Japan) Ltd.
Marion Merrell Dow K. K.
Minophagen Pharmaceutical Co.
Mitsubishi Kasei Co.
Mochida Pharmaceutical Co., Ltd
Nippon Boehringer Ingelheim Co., Ltd.
Nippon Glaxo Ltd.

Nippon Roche K. K.
Nippon Shoji K. K.
Nippon Upjohn K. K.
Nippon Wellcome K. K.
Nov Co., Ltd.
Ono Pharmaceutical Co., Ltd.
Otsuka Pharmaceuticals Co., Ltd.
Ryokuhu-Kai
Sandoz Pharmaceuticals Ltd.
Sankyo Co., Ltd.
Sansho-Kai
Shionogi Co., Ltd.
Taiho Pharmaceutical Co., Ltd.
Takeda Chemical Industries, Ltd.
Tanabe Seiyaku Co., Ltd.
Tokyo Tanabe Co., Ltd.
Torii & Co., Ltd.
Toyobo Co.
Tsumura Co., Ltd.

THE EDITORS

Biological and Molecular Aspects of Mast Cell
and Basophil Differentiation and Function,
edited by Y. Kitamura, S. Yamamoto, S.J. Galli, and
M.W. Greaves. Raven Press, Ltd., New York © 1995.

1

The Effects of Stem Cell Factor, the Ligand for the c-*kit* Receptor, on Mouse and Human Mast Cell Development, Survival, and Function

Stephen J. Galli*, Mindy Tsai*, Barry K. Wershil*†,
Akihiko Iemura‡, Akikazu Ando‖, See-Ying Tam*,
and John J. Costa*¶

*Departments of Pathology, Beth Israel Hospital and Harvard Medical
School, Boston, MA 02215, ¶Department of Medicine, Beth Israel Hospital and
Harvard Medical School, Boston, MA 02215, the †Combined Program in
Pediatric Gastroenterology, The Children's Hospital and Massachusetts General
Hospital, Harvard Medical School, Boston, MA 02215, U.S.A., the ‡First
Department of Pathology and the ‖Department of Pediatrics, Kurume University
School of Medicine, 67-Asahi-machi, Kurume-shi, Fukuoka, 830, Japan.

Stem cell factor (SCF), the ligand for the receptor (SCFR) that is encoded by the c-*kit* protooncogene, has many important effects in rodent and human mast cell development, survival, and function. SCF can promote mast cell survival by suppressing apoptosis, it can induce mast cell hyperplasia in murine rodents, experimental primates and humans, it can directly induce SCFR-dependent mast cell mediator release, and it can significantly modulate the extent of mast cell activation by FcεRI-dependent mechanisms. In this chapter, we will review some of the important effects of SCF in mast cell biology, focusing primarily on the results of *in vivo* studies and on those issues which currently appear to be of clinical relevance in humans.

THE IDENTIFICATION AND CHARACTERIZATION OF STEM CELL FACTOR

In 1979, Russell [1] reviewed an extensive body of evidence indicating that the abnormal phenotypes of both *W**/*W** and *Sl**/*Sl** mutant mice, which exhibit hypoplastic anemia, lack of skin pigmentation and sterility, reflected problems with either the affected lineages (in the *W* mutants) or the microenvironmental cells that regulate the development or survival of the lineages (in the *Sl* mutants). Accordingly, she proposed that the *W* locus encodes a receptor expressed by the cells in the affected lineages and the *Sl* locus encodes a ligand for that receptor. In 1978 and 1979, Kitamura *et al.* [2, 3] reported that, in addition to their other problems, both *W/W^v* and *Sl/Sl^d* mice virtually lack mature mast cells. This work not only provided compelling evidence for the bone marrow origin of tissue mast cells but also illustrated the profound effects of *W* or *Sl* mutations on the mast cell lineage [2, 3]. In 1988, Chabot *et al.* [4] and Geissler *et al.* [5] reported that *W* is allelic with the c-*kit* protooncogene, a member of the receptor tyrosine kinase III family.

In 1990, in confirmation of Russell's hypothesis, three groups simultaneously reported that the *Sl* locus of the mouse encodes a new growth factor which is a ligand for the c-kit receptor [6-8]. This ligand was designated kit ligand [6], mast cell growth factor [7], or stem cell factor (SCF) [8]. Moreover, the latter study demonstrated that injection of recombinant SCF (rSCF) *in vivo* repaired both the anemia and, locally, the mast cell deficiency of *Sl/Sl^d* mice. Subsequently, Geissler *et al.* [9] and Anderson *et al.* [10] mapped the location of the *SCF* gene in humans to chromosome 12, in a linkage group which is highly conserved between humans and mice, and Yasuda *et al.* [11] cloned and functionally characterized the mouse c-*kit* promoter.

The gene for stem cell factor encodes two transmembrane proteins of 220 or 248 amino acids, which are generated by alternative splicing and which may be proteolytically cleaved to produce soluble forms of the molecule which retain biological activity and which spontaneously form non-covalently linked dimers in solution [reviewed in 12]. While the naturally occurring SCF is glycosylated, the non-glycosylated *E. coli*-derived soluble rSCF[164], which was used in most of the studies which we will review herein, has significant biological activity [reviewed in 12].

EFFECTS OF SCF IN MAST CELL DEVELOPMENT AND SURVIVAL

SCF has many effects in mast cell development and function. SCF can maintain mast cell survival by suppressing apoptosis, promote chemotaxis or haptotaxis of mast cells and their precursors, promote the proliferation of immature or mature mast cells, promote the maturation of mast cell precursors or immature mast cells and alter the phenotype and mediator content of these cells, directly promote the degranulation and secretion of mediators by mast cells, enhance the mast cell's ability to secrete mediators in response to other signals, including IgE and specific antigen [reviewed in 12], and alter the expression of other receptors, including those for extracellular matrix components [13, 14]. Moreover, many, perhaps all of these effects of SCF can be modulated by other microenvironmental factors. For example, Tsai *et al.* [15] reported that the administration of recombinant rat SCF to normal rats resulted in the hyperplasia of mast cells in multiple organs, but that the pattern of expression of mast cell-associated proteases by these cells varied in different organs and was appropriate for the specific anatomical sites analyzed. Subsequently, work by Gurish *et al.* [16] in mice, and later by Haig *et al.* [17] in rats, showed that IL-3 not only can augment the ability of SCF to promote mast cell proliferation (an effect previously demonstrated by others, refs. 18, 19) but also can interfere with certain effects of SCF on mast cell protease phenotype.

FIGURE 1. **Numbers of Dermal or Splenic Mast Cells at Various Intervals After Cessation of Chronic Treatment with Recombinant Rat SCF[164] (SCF) in WCB6F$_1$-Sl/Sl^d or -+/+ Mice**

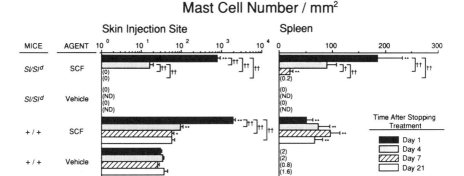

Numbers of mast cells in the dermis at skin injection sites, or in spleen parenchyma, of WCB6F$_1$-Sl/Sl^d (Sl/Sl^d) mice or the congenic normal (+/+) mice which had been injected daily for 3 wk with SCF (100 µg/kg/day) or vehicle. The mice were killed for morphometric quantification of mast cells 1, 4, 7 or 21 days after the last injection of SCF or vehicle. Numbers in parentheses are the mean numbers of mast cells at the indicated intervals. ND, not done.

* p<0.05 and **p<0.01 by the Student's t test, 2-tailed vs. values for corresponding anatomical site in vehicle-injected mice of the same genotype which were killed on the same day after stopping treatment.

† p<0.05 and †† p<0.01 vs. values for the same anatomical site in mice of the same genotype and treatment status which were killed at a different interval after stopping treatment.

Reproduced from ref. 22, *Am J Pathol* 1994;144:321-8, with permission.

SCF PROMOTES MAST CELL SURVIVAL BY SUPPRESSING APOPTOSIS

While all of these effects of SCF are of interest, none of them can be expressed unless the survival of the lineage is maintained. Studies in Sl/Sl^d mice [8, 15] and in cynomolgous monkeys [20] demonstrated that rSCF can promote the survival of the mast cell lineage *in vivo*. Subsequently, two studies established that SCF promotes mast cell survival by suppressing apoptosis. Mekori *et al.* [21] showed that SCF can suppress apoptosis in IL-3-dependent mouse mast cells which are withdrawn from IL-3 *in vitro*. Taking a different approach, Iemura *et al.* [22] showed that SCF can suppress the apoptosis which develops in SCF-dependent mast cells upon withdrawal of the cytokine either *in vitro* or *in vivo*. As shown in Figure 1, SCF treatment (100 µg of recombinant rat SCF/kg/day, s.c., for 21 days) produced a profound cutaneous mast cell hyperplasia in the normal (WCB6F$_1$-+/+) mice, increasing skin mast cell density to ~50-fold that at baseline, and also resulted in the appearance of many mast cells in the skin of WCB6F$_1$-Sl/Sl^d mice, which ordinarily lack both mature mast cells [3] and mast cell precursors in the skin [23]. However, in both WCB6F$_1$-+/+ and -Sl/Sl^d mice, cutaneous mast cell densities rapidly fell to baseline levels within 4 days of cessation of SCF treatment. Histological analysis demonstrated that mast cells at these sites underwent apoptosis upon withdrawal of SCF, but that this process was associated with remarkably little histological evidence of inflammation. The results in the spleens were different in one respect: in the normal (+/+) mice, markedly elevated mast cell densities were retained for at least 21 days after the cessation of SCF treatment. This result indicates that the extent to which the withdrawal of exogenous SCF results in the rapid resolution of SCF-induced mast cell hyperplasia in mice may vary according to anatomical site.

These and other findings in our study showed that mouse mast cells die rapidly by apoptosis after the withdrawal of exogenous SCF either *in vitro* or in most anatomical sites *in vivo*, and indicated that apoptosis represents a mechanism which can account for striking and rapid reductions in the sizes of mast cell populations *in vivo*, such as during development, some immune responses and certain pathological processes, without significant associated inflammation. We also suggested that the increased numbers of mast cells present in mast cell neoplasms or mastocytosis may in part reflect enhanced mast cell survival. We are exploring this issue further and have recently demonstrated that the protooncogene *Bcl-2*, which encodes a product that suppresses apoptosis by promoting an anti-oxidant pathway [24], is overexpressed in a growth factor-independent and tumorigenic mouse mast cell line [25]. However, we also find that certain populations of mast cells can develop in Bcl-2 null mice, a result which indicates that Bcl-2 is not required for the survival of at least some mouse mast cell populations [25].

SCF REGULATES MAST CELL SECRETORY FUNCTION AND MEDIATOR RELEASE

In light of the phenotypic abnormalities expressed by *W* or *Sl* mutant mice, some of the actions of SCF in mast cell biology, such as its ability to suppress apoptosis, might have been considered predictable. However, the cell lineages which are most profoundly affected by *W* or *Sl* mutations are essentially missing in the *W**/*W** or *Sl**/*Sl** mutant animals. Accordingly, it would have been difficult to anticipate that SCF could significantly influence the secretory function of cells which express the SCF receptor. To explore this possibility, we first tested mouse mast cell populations *in vitro*, and showed that relatively high concentrations of SCF could induce mediator release from some mouse mast cells [26]. To investigate the biological significance of this observation, Wershil *et al.* [27] injected SCF or vehicle intradermally into normal WBB6F$_1$-+/+ or WCB6F$_1$-+/+ mice, genetically mast cell-deficient WBB6F$_1$-*W/W^v* or WCB6F$_1$-*Sl/Sl^d* mice, *W/W^v* mice that had been selectively repaired of their cutaneous mast cell deficiency by the adoptive transfer of normal (WBB6F$_1$-+/+) mast cells, which expressed the wild type SCF receptor, and *W/W^v* mice that had been treated with PMA to induce the local development of cutaneous mast cells that expressed the mutant *W^v* SCF receptor [28], which expresses markedly diminished levels of tyrosine kinase activity [29]. This work showed that SCF can induce mouse skin mast cell degranulation *in vivo* in doses as low as 140 fmol/site and that this response is SCF receptor-dependent, in that it occurs when mast cells express the wild type SCF receptor but not the W^v mutant receptor. Notably, dermal mast cells of PMA-treated W/W^v mice exhibited apparently normal degranulation in response to challenge via the $Fc_\varepsilon RI$, a finding which indicates that these cells do not express a generalized impairment of secretory function [27, 28]. Subsequently, it was shown that SCF can also induce mediator release from rat [30] or mouse [31] peritoneal mast cells and from human skin mast cells [32] *in vitro*. At even lower concentrations *in vitro*, SCF can augment IgE-dependent activation of mouse peritoneal mast cell [31] or of human lung [33] or skin [32] mast cells.

The finding that a major regulator of mast cell development also promoted mast cell mediator secretion was both unexpected and provocative. And there were other findings that indicated that signaling of mast cells through the SCFR, a receptor tyrosine kinase, and the $Fc_\varepsilon RI$, a multisubunit receptor with 7 membrane spanning regions but no intrinsic tyrosine kinase activity [34, 35], exhibited certain interesting similarities. Thus, triggering mast cells via either receptor resulted in similar changes in levels of intracellular free Ca++ [32], induced similar patterns of changes in steady state levels of mRNA for early response genes [36], and promoted similar patterns of activation of MAP kinases, pp90^{rsk} and pp70-S6 kinases [37]. On the other hand, the immunosuppressive drug rapamycin inhibited SCFR- or $Fc_\varepsilon RI$-dependent induction of increased activity of pp70-S6 kinase and significantly diminished SCF- or IL-3-dependent mast cell proliferation, but had little or no effect on $Fc_\varepsilon RI$-dependent mast cell mediator release [37]. The latter result suggested either that pp70-S6 kinase activity is not critical for $Fc_\varepsilon RI$-dependent mouse mast cell degranulation, or that the levels of pp70-S6 kinase activity necessary for mast cell mediator release are less than those required for growth-factor-dependent effects on mouse mast cell proliferation.

CHRONIC TREATMENT WITH SCF DOES NOT INCREASE, AND IN SOME CIRCUMSTANCES DIMINISHES, THE INTENSITY OF IGE-DEPENDENT PASSIVE ANAPHYLAXIS IN NORMAL MICE

Given findings indicating that SCF can directly or indirectly enhance mast cell mediator release, and in view of plans to introduce SCF for clinical use, we wondered whether SCF might influence the intensity of IgE-dependent anaphylaxis in genetically mast cell-deficient WCB6F$_1$-*Sl/Sl^d* or congenic normal (WCB6F$_1$-+/+) mice [38]. Accordingly, Ando *et al.* [38] administered rSCF at 100 µg/kg/day subcutaneously or, in control animals, vehicle, daily for 21 days to *Sl/Sl^d* mice and the congenic normal mice. Approximately 4 hours after the last injection of rSCF or vehicle, the mice were passively sensitized with 20 µg of monoclonal mouse IgE anti-DNP antibody given intravenously. One day later, the mice were challenged intravenously with antigen (DNP$_{30-40}$HSA) at 5, 200, or 1000 µg/mouse or, as a control, with saline.

As judged by comparisons with values in the vehicle-treated mice, chronic SCF treatment did not detectably alter "baseline" levels of mast cell degranulation in mice not challenged with antigen. Nor did chronic SCF treatment induce changes in baseline levels of heart rate, pulmonary conductance or pulmonary dynamic compliance (Table I). We found that vehicle-treated *Sl/Sl^d* mice had virtually no tissue mast cells and exhibited neither increased heart rate nor diminished pulmonary conductance or dynamic compliance upon challenge with IgE and antigen. None of the 9 animals tested died. SCF-treated *Sl/Sl^d* mice developed mast cells in multiple tissues, although in most sites the numbers of mast cells were less than those present in the vehicle-treated congenic normal mice. Nevertheless, antigen challenge of these SCF-treated Sl/Sl^d mice produced marked increases in heart rate that were very similar to those seen in identically challenged vehicle- or SCF-treated normal mice. The SCF-treated Sl/Sl^d mice also exhibited reduced dynamic compliance after antigen challenge, although of a lesser magnitude than was seen in the identically challenged +/+ mice. The anaphylactic reactions in SCF-treated Sl/Sl^d mice were associated with extensive mast cell degranulation, but none of the 9 mice in this group died.

Table I.   Effects of Chronic Treatment with Recombinant Rat SCF[164] (SCF, 100 μg/kg/day, s.c., for 21 days) or Vehicle on Tissue Mast Cell Numbers and on the Changes in Heart Rate (HR), Pulmonary Conductance and Dynamic Compliance (G_L, Cdyn), Mast Cell Degranulation, and Death Rates Associated with IgE-Dependent Passive Anaphylaxis in WCB6F$_1$-Sl/Sl^d or -+/+ Mice[†]

Mice	Treatment (21 days)	Mast Cell Numbers	↑HR	↓G_L/Cdyn	Mast Cell Degranulation	Death Rate
Sl/Sl^d	Vehicle	0	0	0	-	0/9
Sl/Sl^d	SCF*	+	+++	+ (Cdyn)	+++	0/9
+/+	Vehicle	++	+++	+++	+++	8/11
+/+	SCF*	+++	+++	+++	+++/+	1/11

[†]   Results are from mice that were challenged with 1000 μg of antigen (DNP$_{30-40}$HSA) on day 22. Note that challenge with vehicle (i.v.) induced no physiological changes, mast cell degranulation or deaths.
*   Chronic SCF treatment (s.c.) did not induce detectable alterations in "baseline" mast cell degranulation or changes in baseline HR, G_L, or Cdyn.
This is a summary of data from ref. 38, reproduced from the *J Clin Invest* 1993;92:1639-49, by copyright permission of the American Society for Clinical Investigation.

Vehicle-treated +/+ mice with normal numbers of tissue mast cells exhibited marked increases in heart rate and decreases in pulmonary conductance and dynamic compliance, as well as extensive mast cell degranulation, upon antigen challenge. And 8 of the 11 animals challenged with the highest dose of antigen died. SCF treatment of normal mice increased mast cell numbers. For example, in the heart and respiratory tract, mast cell numbers were increased 2-3-fold over those in the vehicle treated animals. However the physiological changes produced upon antigen challenge were very similar to those observed in the vehicle-treated animals. In most sites, the extent of mast cell degranulation produced by antigen challenge in the SCF-treated normal mice was essentially the same as that as seen in the vehicle-treated normal mice. However, in the cutaneous SCF injection site, the extent of mast cell degranulation induced at any of the three doses of antigen challenge in the SCF-treated mice actually was significantly <u>less</u> than that at the same dose of antigen challenge in the vehicle-treated normal mice. For example, at 1000 μg of DNP-HSA, 99 ± 0.3% of mast cells exhibited extensive degranulation in the vehicle-treated mice vs. $11 \pm 3\%$ in the SCF-treated mice. And, most remarkably, only 1 of the 11 SCF-treated normal mice died as a result of passive anaphylaxis, a proportion which was significantly less ($p < 0.01$) than that in the identically challenged SCF-treated +/+ mice. In contrast to the results at the highest dose of antigen (1000 µg/mouse), challenge with 200 µg of DNP-HSA produced statistically indistinguishable fatality rates in SCF- vs. vehicle-treated +/+ mice (4/7 vs. 3/8, respectively).

Finally, we repeated the experiments at the highest dose of antigen challenge in +/+ or *Sl/Sl^d* mice that had received the last injection of SCF or vehicle on day 22, one hour (as opposed to one day) before antigen challenge. The results were quite similar to those obtained in mice challenged one day after the last injection of SCF or vehicle: only 1/4 SCF-treated, but 3/5 vehicle-treated, +/+ mice died as a result of passive anaphylaxis; none of the SCF- or vehicle-treated *Sl/Sl^d* mice died.

EFFECTS OF SCF IN EXPERIMENTAL PRIMATES AND HUMANS *IN VIVO*

Chronic treatment with recombinant human SCF (rhSCF), subcutaneously, induced significant mast cell hyperplasia in multiple anatomical sites in both baboons (*Papio cynocephalus*) and cynomolgous monkeys (*Macaca fascicularis*) [20]. The effects were especially notable in organs with a vasculature that readily permits rhSCF to pass from the intravascular to the extravascular space, such as the bone marrow, spleen and liver [20]. For example, treatment of cynomolgous monkeys with rhSCF at 100 µg/kg/day for 21 days induced densities of mast cells that were 3-fold those in vehicle-treated monkeys in the dermis at SCF-injection sites, but had no detectable effect on mast cell densities in skin distant from injection sites, or in the heart, lungs, trachea, thymus or stomach. By contrast, these monkeys had levels of mast cells in the bone marrow, liver, and spleen, that were 7-, 20-, or 128-fold those in the corresponding sites in vehicle-treated monkeys.

By 15 days after cessation of rhSCF treatment in cynomolgous monkeys, mast cell densities in most anatomical sites had returned nearly to baseline levels [20]. Moreover, based on clinical evaluation and autopsy examination of the cynomolgous monkeys, neither the rhSCF treatment, the ensuing mast cell hyperplasia, nor the rapid fall in mast cell numbers after cessation of rhSCF treatment resulted in significant clinical toxicity. In addition, these animals did not exhibit clinical evidence of cutaneous mast cell activation at sites of s.c. injection of rhSCF [20].

In a Phase I trial of rhSCF (5-50 µg/kg/day, s.c., for 14 days) in 10 breast cancer patients, subcutaneous injections of rhSCF produced a wheal and flare response at each injection site [39]. Tramission electron microscopic analysis of biopsies of some of these sites indicated that injections of rhSCF were associated with the development of extensive "anaphylactic type" degranulation of cutaneous mast cells [39]. Three patients exhibited distant adverse effects which may have been related to mast cell activation, and were therefore withdrawn from the study. In the 7 patients who completed the 14 day course of treatment, dermal mast cell density at skin sites not directly injected with rhSCF increased by 70% compared to baseline (pretreatment) values (p=0.022) and normalized urine methyl histamine increased by ~50%. This study suggests that humans may be somewhat more sensitive than cynomolgous monkeys to the mast cell hyperplasia-inducing effects of rhSCF, since 21 days of treatment of the cynomolgous monkey with rhSCF at 100 μg/kg/day did not significantly increase dermal mast cell densities at skin sites distant from rhSCF injection sites [20]. Notably, 5 of the 10 patients treated with rhSCF also developed areas of persistent cutaneous hyperpigmentation at rhSCF injection sites [39].

CONCLUDING REMARKS

In summary, a large body of evidence indicates that SCF/SCF receptor interactions are essential for normal mast cell development in mice [reviewed in 12, 40]. SCF/SCFR receptor interactions are also essential for normal mast cell development in rats, in which a c-*kit* mutation (*Ws*) that produces mast cell deficiency (in *Ws/Ws* rats [41]) has recently been described [reviewed in 40]. Recombinant SCF can promote significant mast cell hyperplasia *in vivo* in mice [15], rats [15], baboons [20], cynomolgous monkeys [20], and humans [39], indicating that SCF/SCFR interactions may be critical for mast cell development and survival in many mammalian species, including humans. SCF can regulate mast cell development and numbers through a broad spectrum of effects at multiple stages of mast cell development and by influencing many cellular functions, including adhesion, migration, survival, proliferation, and differentiation/maturation. However, the effects of SCF can be significantly modulated by other microenvironmental factors, including other cytokines.

SCF also can regulate mast cell secretory function, in both mice and humans, by at least two mechanisms. It can modulate the nature or intensity of the secretory response upon activation of the cells through the IgE receptor or by other mechanisms. Notably, *in vitro* [31-33] or *in vivo* [38] evidence indicates that, depending upon the circumstances, SCF can either upregulate [31-33] or downregulate [38] the intensity of signaling through the mast cell IgE receptor. These effects clearly may have relevance to the regulation of mast cell function during immune responses, allergic disorders, and in certain other diseases. SCF can also directly induce the secretion of mast cell mediators [27, 30-32]. This finding raises the possibility that interactions between SCF and its receptor may modulate mast cell secretory function during diseases or other biological responses that result in changes in levels of SCF bioactivity, or even in normal tissues.

We feel that several issues of established or potential clinical importance need to be explored during the next few years. Clearly, efforts will be made to maximize the benefits of rhSCF in promoting hematopoiesis or in facilitating the generation or recovery of hematopoietic progenitor cells, while minimizing any adverse effects associated with the cytokine, such as the induction of mast cell hyperplasia or activation [42]. It also will be important to assess whether rhSCF can be used safely in subjects with allergic diseases or other disorders associated with mast cell activation. In the study by Ando *et al.*, [38] it is not clear whether the ability of chronic treatment with rSCF to reduce fatalities associated with passive anaphylaxis in mice primarily reflected an action of the cytokine on mast cells, as opposed to effects on other cell types which express SCF receptors. Nor can the findings in mice be used to predict the effects of chronic treatment with rhSCF in human subjects. However, our results do raise the possibility that, at least under some circumstances, the administration of rhSCF to patients with allergic diseases may not only be safe, but could even confer benefit. It will also be of interest to determine whether interfering with mast cell survival, for example by blocking SCF receptor-dependent suppression of apoptosis, can have clinical benefit in certain settings. Finally, we are sure that additional uses of rhSCF will be explored, based on the effects of this cytokine on other lineages that express the stem cell factor receptor, such as melanocytes and germ cells.

ACKNOWLEDGMENTS

The work reviewed herein was supported by United States Public Health Service grants, the Beth Israel Hospital Pathology Foundation, Inc., and AMGEN, Inc. SJG and JJC perform research funded by, and consult for, AMGEN, Inc., under terms that are in accord with Beth Israel Hospital and Harvard Medical School conflict of interest policies.

REFERENCES

1. Russell ES. Hereditary anemias of the mouse: a review for geneticists. *Adv Genetics* 1979;20:357-459.
2. Kitamura Y, Go S, Hatanaka S. Decrease of mast cells in *W/Wv* mice and their increase by bone marrow transplantation. *Blood* 1978;52:447-52.
3. Kitamura Y, Go S. Decreased production of mast cells in *Sl/Sld* mice. *Blood* 1979;53:492-7.
4. Chabot B, Stephenson DA, Chapman VM, Besmer P, Bernstein A. The protooncogene c-*kit* encoding a transmembrane tyrosine kinase receptor maps to the mouse *W* locus. *Nature* 1988;355:88-9.
5. Geissler EN, Ryan MA, Housman DE. The dominant-white spotting (*W*) locus of the mouse encodes the c-*kit* protooncogene. *Cell* 1988;55:185-92.
6. Huang E, Nocka K, Beier DR, Chu T-Y, Buck J, Lahm H-W, et al. The hematopoietic growth factor KL is encoded at the *Sl* locus and is the ligand of the c-*kit* receptor, the gene product of the *W* locus. *Cell* 1990;63:225-33.
7. Williams DE, Eisenman J, Baird A, Rauch C, van Ness K, March CJ, et al. Identification of a ligand for the c-*kit* protooncogene. *Cell* 1990;63:167-74.
8. Zsebo KM, Williams DA, Geissler EN, Broudy VC, Martin FH, Atkins HL, et al. Stem cell factor (SCF) is encoded at the *Sl* locus of the mouse and is the ligand for the c-kit tyrosine kinase receptor. *Cell* 1990;63:213-24.
9. Geissler EN, Liao M, Brook JD, Martin FH, Zsebo KM, Housman DE, et al. Stem Cell Factor (*SCF*), a novel hematopoietic growth factor and a ligand for the c-kit tyrosine kinase receptor, maps on human chromosome 12 between 12q14.3 and 12qter. *Som Cell Mol Gen* 1991;17:207-14.
10. Anderson DM, Williams DE, Tushinski R, et al. Alternate splicing of mRNAs encoding human mast cell growth factor and localization of the gene to chromosome 12q22-q24. *Cell Growth Differ* 1991;2:373-8.
11. Yasuda H, Galli SJ, Geissler EN. Cloning and functional analysis of the mouse c-*kit* promoter. *Biochem Biophys Res Comm* 1993;191:893-901.
12. Galli SJ, Zsebo KM, Geissler EN. The kit ligand, stem cell factor. *Adv Immunol* 1994;55:1-96.
13. Dastych J, Metcalfe DD. Stem cell factor induces mast cell adhesion to fibronectin. *J Immunol* 1994;152:213-9.
14. Kinashi T, Springer TA. Steel factor and c-*kit* regulate cell-matrix adhesion. *Blood* 1994;83:1033-8.

15. Tsai M, Shih L-S, Newlands GFJ, et al. The rat *c-kit* ligand, stem cell factor, induces the development of connective tissue-type and mucosal mast cells *in vivo*. Analysis by anatomical distribution, histochemistry and protease phenotype. *J Exp Med* 1991;174:125-31.
16. Gurish MF, Ghildyal N, McNeil HP, Austen KF, Gillis S, Stevens RL. Differential expression of secretory granule proteases in mouse mast cells exposed to interleukin 3 and c-*kit* ligand. *J Exp Med* 1992;175:1003-12.
17. Haig DM, Huntley JF, MacKellar A, Newlands GFJ, Inglis L, Sangha R, et al. Effects of stem cell factor (kit-ligand) and interleukin-3 on the growth and serine proteinase expression of rat bone marrow-derived or serosal mast cells. *Blood* 1994;83:72-83.
18. Tsuji K, Zsebo KM, Ogawa M. Murine mast cell colony formation supported by IL-3, IL-4, and recombinant rat stem cell factor, ligand for c-kit. *J Cell Physiol* 1991;148:362-9.
19. Takagi M, Nakahata T, Kubo T, et al. Stimulation of mouse connective tissue-type mast cells by hemopoietic stem cell factor, a ligand for the c-*kit* receptor. *J Immunol* 1992;148:3446-53.
20. Galli SJ, Iemura A, Garlick DS, Gamba-Vitalo C, Zsebo KM, Andrews RG. Reversible expansion of primate mast cell populations *in vivo* by stem cell factor. *J Clin Invest* 1993;91:148-52.
21. Mekori YA, Oh CK, Metcalfe DD. IL-3-dependent murine mast cells undergo apoptosis on removal of IL-3. Prevention of apoptosis by c-*kit* ligand. *J Immunol* 1993;151:3775-84.
22. Iemura A, Tsai M, Ando A, Wershil BK, Galli SJ. The c-*kit* ligand, stem cell factor, promotes mast cell survival by suppressing apoptosis. *Am J Pathol* 1994;144:321-8.
23. Hayashi C, Sonoda T, Nakano T, Nakayama H, Kitamura Y. Mast cell precursors in the skin of mouse embryos and their deficiency in embryos of *Sl/Sl*^{d} genotype. *Dev Biol* 1985;109:234-41.
24. Hockenberry DM, Oltvai ZN, Yin X-M, Millman CL, Korsmeyer SJ. Bcl-2 functions in an antioxidant pathway to prevent apoptosis. *Cell* 1993;75:241-51.
25. Tsai M, Tam S-Y, Veis DJ, Korsmeyer SJ, Galli SJ. Bcl-2 and mast cell survival: Bcl-2 is overexpressed in a growth factor-independent mouse mast cell line but mast cells develop in Bcl-2 null mice. *FASEB J* 1994;8:A742.
26. Galli SJ, Tsai M, Langley KE, Zsebo KM, Geissler EN. Stem cell factor (SCF), a ligand for *c-kit*, induces mediator release from some populations of mouse mast cells. *FASEB J* 1991;5:A1092.
27. Wershil BK, Tsai M, Geissler EN, Zsebo KM, Galli SJ. The rat *c-kit* ligand, stem cell factor, induces c-*kit* receptor-dependent mouse mast cell activation *in vivo*. Evidence that signaling through the c-*kit* receptor can induce expression of cellular function. *J Exp Med* 1992;175:245-55.
28. Gordon JR, Galli SJ. Phorbol 12-myristate 13-acetate-induced development of functionally active mast cells in *W/W*^{v} but not *Sl/Sl*^{d} genetically mast cell-deficient mice. *Blood* 1990;75:1637-45.
29. Nocka K, Tan J, Chiu E, et al. Molecular bases of dominant negative and loss of function mutations at the murine c-*kit*/white spotting locus: W^{37}, W^v, W^{41} and W. *EMBO J* 1990;9:1805-13.
30. Nakajima K, Hirai K, Yamaguchi M, Takaishi T, Ohta K, Morita Y, et al. Stem cell factor has histamine releasing activity in rat connective tissue-type mast cells. *Biochem Biophys Res Commun* 1992;183:1076-83.

31. Coleman JW, Holliday MR, Kimber I, Zsebo KM, Galli SJ. Regulation of mouse peritoneal mast cell secretory function by stem cell factor, IL-3 or IL-4. *J Immunol* 1993;150:556-62.

32. Columbo M, Horowitz EM, Botana LM, MacGlashan DW Jr, Bochner BS, Gillis S, et al. The human recombinant *c-kit* receptor ligand, rhSCF, induces mediator release from human cutaneous mast cells and enhances IgE-dependent mediator release from both skin mast cells and peripheral blood basophils. *J Immunol* 1992;149:599-608.

33. Bischoff SC, Dahinden CA. c-*kit* ligand: a unique potentiator of mediator release by human lung mast cells. *J Exp Med* 1992;175:237-44.

34. Kinet JP. The gamma-zeta dimers of Fc receptors as connectors to signal transduction. *Curr Opin Today* 1993;14:43-8.

35. Beaven MA, Metzger H. Signal trnasuction by Fc receptor: the Fc epsilon RI case. *Immunol Today* 1993;14:222-6.

36. Tsai M, Tam S-Y, Galli SJ. Distinct patterns of early response gene expression and proliferation in mouse mast cells stimulated by stem cell factor, interleukin-3, or IgE and antigen. *Eur J Immunol* 1993;23:867-72.

37. Tsai M, Chen R-H, Tam S-Y, Blenis J, Galli SJ. Activation of MAP kinases, pp90^{rsk} and pp70-S6 kinases in mouse mast cells by signaling through the c-*kit* receptor tyrosine kinase or Fc$_\varepsilon$RI: Rapamycin inhibits activation of pp70-S6 kinase and proliferation in mouse mast cells. *Eur J Immunol* 1993;23:3286-91.

38. Ando A, Martin TR, Galli SJ. Effects of chronic treatment with the c-kit ligand, stem cell factor, on immunoglobulin E-dependent anaphylaxis in mice: Genetically mast cell-deficient *Sl/Sl^d* mice acquire anaphylactic responsiveness, but the congenic normal mice do not exhibit augmented responses. *J Clin Invest* 1993;92:1639-49.

39. Costa JJ, Demetri GD, Harrist TJ, Dvorak AM, Hayes DF, Merica EA, et al. Recombinant human stem cell factor (rhSCF) induces cutaneous mast cell activation and hyperplasia, and hyperpigmentation in humans *in vivo*. *J Allergy Clin Immunol* 1994;93:225 (abstr).

40. Kitamura Y, Tsujimura T, Jippo T, Nomura S. Regulation of development, survival and neoplastic growth of mast cells through c-kit receptor. *Int Archs Allergy Immunol*, in press.

41. Niwa Y, Kasugai T, Ohno K, et al. Anemia and mast cell depletion in mutant rats that are homozygous at "white spotting *(Ws)*" locus. *Blood* 1991;78:1936-41.

42. Morstyn GS, Brown S, Gordon M, et al. Stem cell factor is a potent synergistic factor in hematopoiesis. *Oncology* 1994;51:205-14.

Biological and Molecular Aspects of Mast Cell
and Basophil Differentiation and Function,
edited by Y. Kitamura, S. Yamamoto, S.J. Galli, and
M.W. Greaves. Raven Press, Ltd., New York © 1995.

2

Synergy of stem cell factor and other cytokines in mast cell development

Tatsutoshi Nakahata, Kohichiro Tsuji, Ryuhei Tanaka, Kenji Muraoka, Nobuo Okumura[1], Nobukuni Sawai[2], Mineo Takagi[2], Susumu Itoh[3], Chisei Ra[4], Hirohisa Saito[5]

Department of Clinical Oncology, Institute of Medical Science, University of Tokyo, Tokyo 108, Japan

[1]*Division of Clinical Chemistry and Medical Technology, School of Allied Medical Sciences,*

[2]*Department of Pediatrics and* [3]*Department of Blood Transfusion, Shinshu University School of Medicine, Matsumoto 390, Japan*

[4]*Department of Immunology, Juntendo University School of Medicine, Tokyo 113, Japan*

[5]*Division of Allergy, National Children's Medical Research Center, Tokyo 154, Japan*

Mast cell precursors are derived from multipotential hematopoietic stem cells, migrate in the bloodstream, and enter the tissues where they differentiate into morphologically identifiable mast cells (1). The differentiated mast cells may be classified into at least two phenotypically distinct subpopulations in rodents; connective tissue-type mast cells (CTMC) and mucosal mast cells (MMC) (2), and in human; tryptase[+] chymase[-] mast cell (T mast) and tryptase[+] chymase[+] mast cell (TC mast) (3). Several investigators reported a further subclass of murine mast cells (BMMC) which arise when normal mouse hematopoietic cells are cultured with IL-3 (4, 5). It has been thought that the IL-3-dependent BMMC are tissue culture equivalents of the MMC subclass, since the cells stain with alcian blue but not with safranin or berberine sulfate, a cationic fluorescent dye that binds to the sulfate

13

containing-polyanions in heparin, as do MMC. However, recent studies of mast cell protease mRNAs demonstrated that mouse BMMC are very immature CTMC (6, 7).

In contrast to the situation in the murine system, IL-3 apparently is no growth or differentiation factor for human mast cells in culture of bone marrow cells (8). Recently, a gene encoding the ligand for c-kit was cloned by several groups (9-11), and named stem cell factor (SCF) (12), mast cell growth factor (MGF) (10), or kit ligand growth factor (KL) (11). More recently, several investigators reported that the growth of human mast cells was successfully induced in long term cultures of bone marrow cells or cord blood cells by the use of SCF (13, 14). However, a growth factor other than SCF for human mast cells and synergistic factors in conjunction with SCF for both murine and human mast cells remained to be elucidated. The present paper describes the effects of SCF on the growth of murine and human mast cells from hemopoietic progenitors in the presence of other cytokines.

I. EFFECTS OF SCF ON THE GROWTH OF MURINE BMMC

First we have examined the effects of stem cell factor in combination with other cytokines on the proliferation of mouse BMMC. BMMC were prepared by pooling pure mast cell colonies which were obtained from the secondary cultures of blast cell colonies with IL-3 (15). The blast cell colonies were cultured with IL-3 from bone marrow cells of mice which had been injected with 150 mg/kg 5-fluorouracil (5-FU) through the tail vein 2 days before marrow harvest, as described previously (16). All of BMMC stain with alcian blue but not with safranin. Methylcellulose culture was carried out using a modification of a technique described previously (17, 18). One milliliter of culture mixture containing 5×10^2 mouse BMMC, α-medium, 1.2% methylcellulose, 30% fetal bovine serum (FBS), 1% deionized bovine serum albumin (BSA), 1×10^{-4} M 2-mercaptoethanol (2-ME) and cytokines (IL-3, IL-4, SCF) was plated in 35 mm Lux standard nontissue culture dishes. The dishes were incubated at 37°C in a humidified atmosphere flushed with 5% CO_2. Mast cell colonies containing 20 or more cells were scored on an inverted microscope on day 14 of culture. Mouse recombinant IL-3, IL-4 and rat recombinant SCF were used at concentrations of 10 ng/ml, 10 ng/ml and 25 ng/ml , respectively.

Table 1 shows the result of the culture of BMMC with various combinations of IL-3, IL-4 and SCF. IL-3 alone supported the colony formation from BMMC, while IL-4 or SCF did not by themselves. Addition of IL-4 to the culture with IL-3 significantly increased mast cell colony number. SCF also enhanced the IL-3 dependent colony formation, but, interestingly, 25 ng/ml SCF supported more colonies than 100 ng/ml SCF in the presence of IL-3. Although IL-4 or SCF alone could not support any colony growth, a combination of IL-4 and SCF synergistically induced mast cell colony formation from BMMC. The combination of the three factors, IL-3, IL-4 and SCF induced the largest number of mast cell colonies, but 25 ng/ml SCF again supported more colonies than 100 ng/ml SCF.

Table 1. Effects of SCF on mast cell colony formation from BMMC

Factors				Number of mast cell colonies/500 BMMC
IL-3 (200U/ml)	IL-4 (10ng/ml)	SCF (25ng/ml)	SCF (100ng/ml)	
+	-	-	-	56±5
-	+	-	-	0
-	-	+	-	0
-	-	-	+	0
+	+	-	-	100±1
+	-	+	-	76±6
+	-	-	+	64±4
-	+	+	-	85±4
-	+	-	+	85±3
+	+	+	-	121±7
+	+	-	+	89±5

To examine the effects of SCF on mast cell colony formation from BMMC in more detail, we carried out dose response experiments of SCF (data not shown). SCF augmented the IL-3-dependent mast cell colony formation dose-dependently and reached a maximal level at a concentration of 25 ng/ml. Higher concentrations of SCF acted inhibitory. SCF also induced mast cell colony formation dose-dependently in the presence of IL-4 and reached a plateau level at a concentration of 25 ng/ml SCF. In contrast with the culture with IL-3, higher concentrations of SCF did not inhibited the colony formation. The mechanism of inhibitory effect of SCF in the case of IL-3-containing culture is now being studied. The preliminary result of cytochemical examination has shown that a part of mast cells in the colonies supported by SCF stain with safranin and berberine sulfate. This result suggests the possibility that SCF may induce not only the proliferation of BMMC but also phenotypical change of BMMC to CTMC.

II. SCF STIMULATES THE GROWTH OF BMMC IN THE PRESENCE OF IL-10

IL-10 was initially detected as a cytokine produced by Th2 cells that inhibited production of cytokines by Th1 cells, and cDNA clones encoding mouse IL-10 were isolated from cDNA library of Con A-stimulated Th2 clones (19). It was reported that IL-10 stimulates the growth of MC/9 mast cell line and mast cell precursors in mouse mesenteric lymph node cells (20), and induces transcription of the genes for MMCP-1 and 2 in BMMC (21, 22). However, little are known about the action of IL-10 on the proliferation of BMMC. Then we have now examined the effects of IL-10 alone or in combinations with other cytokines including SCF on the growth of BMMC using a methylcellulose culture method. Table 2 shows the mast cell colony formation from BMMC by 10 ng/ml IL-10 in combinations with IL-3, IL-4 or SCF. IL-10 alone did not induce the mast cell colony formation, but IL-10 enhanced the IL-3-dependent mast cell colony formation. Although SCF, IL-4 or IL-10 alone failed to support any colony growth, combinations of IL-4 + IL-10 and SCF + IL-10 synergistically induced mast cell colony formation from BMMC. This result indicates that IL-10 has synergistic action with IL-3, IL-4 or SCF in the proliferation of BMMC. To confirm the synergistic action of IL-10, we carried out dose response experiments. In all of the three cases (IL-3 + IL-10, IL-4 + IL-10 and SCF + IL-10) IL-10 induced mast cell colony formation dose-dependently. These results indicate that

IL-10 also plays an important role in the development of BMMC.

Table 2. Effects of IL-10 on the growth of BMMC

Factors	No of colonies / 5×10^2 BMMC
None	0
IL-10	0
IL-3	28 ± 1
IL-10 + IL-3	43 ± 0
IL-4	0
IL-10 + IL-4	69 ± 2
SCF	0
IL-10 + SCF	29 ± 4

In summary of mouse studies, all the findings presented here indicate that the development of BMMC is regulated by interaction of various cytokines including SCF, IL-3, IL-4 and IL-10.

III. SCF IN COMBINATION WITH IL-6 OR IL-11 SIGNIFICANTLY STIMULATED GENERATION OF HUMAN MAST CELLS FROM CORD BLOOD MNC

Next we examined the effects of SCF on the development of human mast cells. Human umbilical cord blood, collected according to institutional guidance, were obtained during normal full-term deliveries. Mononuclear cells (MNC) were separated by Ficoll-Hypaque density gradient centrifugation after depletion of phagocytes with Silica (23). MNC were incubated in suspension culture using a modification of the techniques as described previously (24, 25). Ten milliliter of culture mixture containing 1×10^6 MNC/ml, α-medium, 20% FBS, 1% BSA and different combinations of cytokines was incubated in 50 ml-tissue plates at 37° C in a humidified atmosphere flushed with 5% CO_2. At weekly intervals, cultures were demi-depopulated by the removal of half the culture volume, which was then replaced by newly-prepared medium with same combinations of cytokines. Cells in the collected media were washed, counted and stained. All the cytokines were pure recombinant molecules and were used at concentrations that induced optimal response in methylcellulose culture of human hemopoietic cells.

When we cultured cord blood MNC in the presence of more than 100 ng/ml human SCF alone a few mast cells were detected after 3 weeks of culture. Other cytokines including IL-1, IL-2, IL-3, IL-4, IL-5, IL-6, IL-7, IL-11, IL-13, G-CSF, GM-CSF, M-CSF, EPO and ligand for flk2 alone or combinations failed to support generation of any mast cells. In contrast, combinations of SCF and IL-6 or IL-11, but not SCF, IL-6 or IL-11 alone were found to dramatically stimulate generation of human mast cells from cord blood MNC (Fig. 1). To confirm the nature of human mast cells, monoclonal antibody reaction against human tryptase were detected using the alkaline phosphatase anti-alkaline phosphatase (APAAP) method (26). Mast cells with tryptase-positive granules were first detected after 2 weeks of culture with SCF and IL-6 or IL-11, increased dramatically and reached to almost 90 % purity after 67 days of culture with SCF and IL-6 (Fig. 1 and 2).

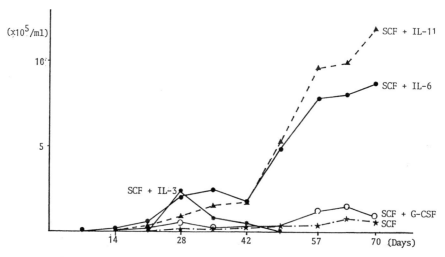

Fig. 1   Generation of mast cells from human cord blood MNC in culture
with SCF and IL-6 or IL-11

Interestingly, addition of IL-3 or GM-CSF to culture with SCF alone or in combination with IL-6 or IL-11 significantly inhibited the mast cell production (Fig. 1 and 2).

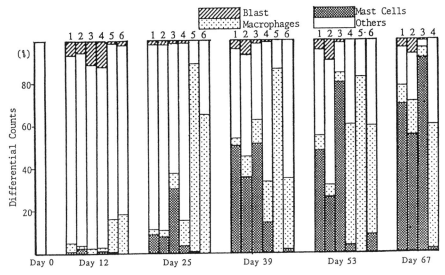

1:SCF, 2:SCF+IL-11, 3:SCF+IL-6, 4:SCF+IL-3, 5:SCF+GM-CSF, 6:SCF+IL-3+GM-CSF

Fig 2. Development of human mast cells from CB MNC
(differential cell counts)

These findings demonstrated that SCF is a most important factor for the generation of human mast cells and IL-6 or IL-11 could stimulate it in conjunction with SCF, suggesting that the mast cell progenitors in cord blood MNC are responsive to signalling through c-kit receptor as well as gp130 which is a signal transducing receptor component utilized in common by receptor complexes for IL-6 and IL-11 (27).

IV. A COMBINATION OF SCF AND IL-6 SUPPORTED GENERATION OF HUMAN MAST CELLS FROM CORD BLOOD CD34+ CELLS

Next we examined the effect of SCF in conjunction with IL-6 or IL-11 on the development of human mast cells from purified CD34$^+$ cells. We used an immunomagnetic system for the purification of CD34$^+$ cells. In brief, MNC were mixed with Dynabeads M-450 CD34 (Dynal, Oslo, Norway), with a bead to cell ratio of 1:1. Cell-beads suspension was resuspended well and incubated at 4° C for 30 minutes. Dynabeads M-450 CD 34/rosetted cells were collected in a Dynal MPC (Magnetic Particle Concentrator) and beads were detached by DETACH HaBead CD34 (Dynal) from the positively selected cells. Eighty-five to 95% of the cells separated were CD 34 positive by FACS analysis.

Culture of CD34$^+$ cells in the presence of SCF and IL-6 or IL-11 indicated more efficient generation of human mast cells than the culture of MNC. More than ten million of pure mast cells were obtained by culturing of 20000 CD34$^+$ cells in the presence of SCF and IL-6 at day 120. Fig. 3 shows in situ appearance of our cultured mast cells after 120 days of culture with a combination of SCF and IL-6, indicating homogeneous generation of human mast cells. Immuno-staining with monoclonal antibody against human tryptase revealed that all of the cells, which were harvested from the culture of CD34$^+$ cells in the presence of a combination of SCF and IL-6 at 120 days, were tryptase-positive.

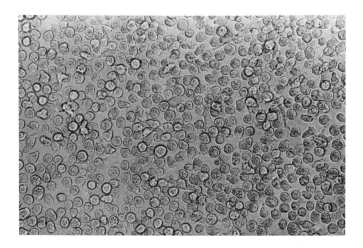

Fig. 3. In situ appearance of human cultured mast cells.

V. GENERATION OF BOTH T AND TC MAST CELLS FROM CORD BLOOD CD34⁺ CELLS IN CULTURE WITH SCF AND IL-6

To confirm whether a combination with SCF and IL-6 could support the generation not only tryptase-positive T mast cells but also tryptase- and chymase double positive TC mast cells, at weekly intervals, a part of culture medium was collected, and cytocentrifuge preparations were made after cell counting and washing 3 times and immuno-stained with anti-human tryptase and anti-human chymase monoclonal antibodies. Weekly analysis of constituent cells in culture of CD34⁺ cells revealed that tryptase-positive cells were first identified at 2 week of culture and chymase-positive cells at 7 weeks. After 100 days of culture, almost 100% of the cells were tryptase positive and 20-30% of the cells were immunologically stained for chymase. These results demonstrated that both T and TC mast cells were induced from CD34⁺ cells in the presence of SCF + IL-6. Our cultured mast cells contained a large amount of histamine and tryptase, expressed functional high affinity IgE receptors, and could proliferate and survive for more than 1 year.

In the present paper, we demonstrated that a combination of SCF and IL-6 is a suitable combination of cytokines for the development of human cultured mast cells from mast cell progenitors in CD34⁺ cell population. Previous reports suggested the dependency of induction and proliferation of human TC mast cells on stroma cells (28). However, our results clearly demonstrated that both T and TC mast call were inducible from CD34⁺ cells in the presence of SCF and IL-6 and in the absence of stromal cells. Our cultured mast cells may provide a novel means to clarify the physiological and pathological characteristics of human mast cells.

ACKNOWLEDGEMENTS

This work was supported in part by grants from Ministry of Education, Science and Culture, Japan. We would like to thank Ms. Ikuko Tanaka for technical support.

REFERENCES

1. Kitamura Y, Sonoda T, Nakano T, Hayashi C, Asai H. Differentiation

processes of connective tissue mast cells in living mice. *Int Arch Allergy Appl Immunol* 1985:77:144-150.

2. Galli SJ, Dvorak AM, Dvorak HF. Basophils and mast cells: morphologic insights into their biology, secretory patterns, and function. *Prog Allergy* 1984: 34:1-141.

3. Schwartz L B. Heterogeneity of human mast cells. In:Kaliner M A, Metcalfe DD. *The mast cell in health and disease.* Marcel Dekker Inc; 1993: 219-236.

4. Nabel G, Galli SJ, Dvorak AM, Dvorak HF, Cantor H. Inducer T lymphocytes synthesize a factor that stimulates proliferation of cloned mast cells. *Nature* 1981:291:332-334.

5. Schrader JW, Lewis SJ, Clark-Lewis I, Culvenor J G. The persistent (P) cell: histamine content, regulation by a T cell-derived factor, origin from a bone marrow precursor, and relationship to mast cells. *Proc Natl Acad Sci USA* 1981: 78:323-327.

6. Serafin WE, Reynolds DS, Rogelj S, et al. Identification and molecular cloning of a novel mouse mucosal mast cell serine protease. *J Biol Chem* 1990: 265:423-429.

7. Reynolds DS, Gurley DS, Austen KF, Serafin WE. Cloning of the cDNA and gene of mouse mast cell protease-6: transcription by progenitor mast cells and mast cells of connective tissue subclass. *J Biol Chem* 1991:266:3847-3853.

8. Saito H, Hatake K, Dvorak A M, et al. Selective differentiation and proliferation of hematopoietic cells induced by recombinant human interleukins. *Proc Natl Acad Sci USA* 1988: 85:2288-2292.

9. Martin FH, Suggs SV, Langley KE, et al. Primary structure and functional expression of rat and human stem cell factor DNAs. *Cell* 1990: 63:203-211.

10. Anderson DM, Lyman SD, Baird A, et al. Molecular cloning of mast cell growth factor, a hematopoietin that is active in both membrane bound and soluble forms. *Cell* 1990: 63:235-243.

11. Huang E, Nocka K, Beier DR, et al. The hematopoietic growth factor KL is encoded by the Sl locus and is the ligand of the c-kit receptor, the gene product of the *W* locus. *Cell* 1990: 63:225-233.

12. Zsebo KM, Wypych J, Mcniece IK, et al. Identification, purification, and biological characterization of hematopoietic stem cell factor from buffalo rat

liver-conditioned medium. *Cell* 1990: 63:195-201.

13. Valent P, Spanbløchl E, Sperr W R, et al. Induction of differentiation of human mast cells from bone marrow and peripheral blood mononuclear cells by recombinant human stem cell factor/kit-ligand in long-term culture. *Blood* 1992: 80:2237-2245.

14. Irani A-M A, Nilsson G, Miettinen U, et al. Recombinant human stem cell factor stimulates differentiation of mast cells from dispersed human fetal liver cells. *Blood* 1992: 80: 3009-3021.

15. Tsuji K, Zsebo KM, Ogawa M. Murine mast cell colony formation supported by IL-3, IL-4, and recombinant rat stem cell factor, ligand for c-kit. *J Cell Physiol* 1991:148:362-369.

16. Koike K, Nakahata T, Takagi M, et al. Synergism of BSF-2/interleukin 6 and interleukin 3 on development of multipotential hemopoietic progenitors in serum-free culture. *J Exp Med* 1988:168:879-890.

17. Nakahata T, Spicer SS, Canty JR, Ogawa M. Clonal assay of mouse mast cell clonies in methylcellulose culture. *Blood* 1982:60:352-361.

18. Nakahata T, Kobayashi T, Ishiguro A, et al. Extensive proliferation of mature connective-tissue type mast cells in vitro. *Nature* 1986:324:65-67.

19. Moore KW, Vieira P, Fiorentino DF, Trounstine ML, Khan TA, Mosmann TR. Homology of cytokine synthesis inhibitory factor (IL-10) to the Epstein Barr Virus gene BCRFI. *Science* 1990:248:1230-1234.

20. Thompson-spipes L, Dhar V, Bond MW, Mosmann TR, Moore KW, Rennick DM. Interleukin 10: A novel stimulatory factor for mast cells and their progenitors. *J Exp Med* 1991:173:507-510.

21. Ghildyal N, McNeil HP, Stechschulte S, et al. IL-10 induces transcription of the gene for mouse mast cell protease-1, a serine protease preferentially expressed in mucosal mast cells of trichinella spiralis-infected mice. *J Immunol* 1992:149:2123-2129.

22. Ghildyal N, McNeil HP, Gurish MF, Austen KF, Stevens RL. Transcriptional regulation of the mucosal mast cell-specific protease gene, MMCP-2, by interleukin 10 and interleukin 3. *J Biol Chem* 1992:267:8473-8477.

23. Imai T, Koike K, Kubo T, et al. Interleukin-6 supports human megakaryocytic proliferation and differentiation in vitro. *Blood* 1991:78:1969-1974.

24. Ogawa M, Nakahata T, Leary A G, Sterk A R , Ishizaka K, Ishizaka T. Suspension culture of human mast cells/basophils from umbilical cord blood mononuclear cells. *Proc Natl Acad Sci USA* 1983:80:4494-4498.

25 Mayani H, Lansdorp P M. Thy-1 expression is linked to functional properties of primitive hematopoietic progenitor cells from human umbilical cord blood. *Blood* 1994:83:2410-2417.

26. Okumura N, Tsuji K, Nakahata T. Change in cell surface antigen expressions during proliferation and differentiation of human erythroid progenitors. *Blood* 1992:80:642-650.

27. Yin T, Taga T, Tsang M L-S, Yasukawa K, Kishimoto T, Yang Y-C. Involvement of IL-6 signal transducer gp130 in IL-11-mediated signal transduction. *J Immunol* 1993: 151: 2555-2561.

28. Furitsu T, Saito H, Dvorak AM, et al. Development of human mast cells in vitro. *Proc Natl Acad Sci USA* 1989: 86: 10039-10043.

Biological and Molecular Aspects of Mast Cell
and Basophil Differentiation and Function,
edited by Y. Kitamura, S. Yamamoto, S.J. Galli, and
M.W. Greaves. Raven Press, Ltd., New York © 1995.

3

Cytokine Regulation of Arachidonic Acid Metabolism in Mast Cells

Makoto Murakami, K. Frank Austen, and Jonathan P. Arm

Department of Medicine, Harvard Medical School, and Department of Rheumatology and Immunology, Brigham and Women's Hospital, Boston, Massachusetts 02115

Mast cells are highly specialized effector cells of the immune system that, when activated, release a diversity of biologically active, granule-associated mediators; produce cytokines; and generate lipid-derived eicosanoids and platelet-activating factor (1). Serosal mast cells, generally studied as a connective tissue mast cell (CTMC) surrogate, respond to Fcε receptor I (FcεRI)-dependent activation with preferred generation of the cyclooxygenase pathway product, prostaglandin (PG) D_2, whereas rat mucosal mast cells (MMC) and mouse bone marrow-derived mast cells (BMMC) developed in interleukin (IL) -3 generate leukotriene (LT) C_4 via the 5-lipoxygenase (5-LO) pathway in preference to PGD_2 (2,3).

The initial step in arachidonic acid metabolism is the release of free arachidonic acid from cell membrane phospholipids by phospholipase A_2 (PLA_2). Prostaglandin endoperoxide synthase (PGHS, or cyclooxygenase), which occurs in two isoforms (PGHS-1 and PGHS-2), directly catalyzes the oxygenation of arachidonic acid to PGG_2, which is reduced to PGH_2 by the hydroperoxidase activity of the same enzyme. PGH_2 is metabolized by specific PG synthases, each of which has a restricted distribution, to individual prostanoids. 5-LO catalyzes the sequential metabolism of arachidonic acid to 5-hydroperoxyeicosatetraenoic acid and then to LTA_4. A perinuclear membrane protein, termed 5-LO activating protein (FLAP), presents arachidonic acid to 5-LO. LTA_4 is processed to LTC_4 by LTC_4 synthase, a perinuclear protein with restricted substrate specificity (Fig. 1).

The tissue-specific elements that direct the appearance of a mast cell phenotype that responds to IgE-mediated activation with preferential generation of PGD_2 or LTC_4 are unknown. Mouse BMMC are capable of differentiating to either phenotype of mature mast cells, CTMC and MMC, depending on the local tissue microenvironment where they reside (4). Two cytokines, c-*kit* ligand (KL, also known as stem cell factor or *steel* factor) and IL-3, can support survival and proliferation of non-transformed mast cells *in vitro* (5-7). KL, a stromal cytokine, elicits differentiation and maturation of BMMC toward a CTMC-like phenotype in terms of granule maturation based upon heparin biosynthesis, increased histamine content, and expression of the CTMC-specific mouse mast cell protease, mMCP-4 (8,9). Various other cytokines, such as IL-1β, IL-4, IL-9, IL-10, nerve growth factor (NGF), transforming growth factor (TGF) β, and interferon (IFN) γ, influence proliferation, differentiation, maturation, survival, chemotaxis, or effector functions of mast cells *in vitro* in combination with IL-3 or KL (10-20).

   In this article, we discuss the regulation of arachidonic acid metabolism in BMMC by hematopoietic cytokines and by a stromal cytokine, KL. KL primes BMMC for increased IgE-dependent production of PGD_2 over several days of culture, thereby eliciting maturation toward the CTMC phenotype (21). KL directly induces PGD_2 generation over several hours of culture, before its priming effect (10). The regulatory mechanisms of these two events at each enzyme step are discussed.

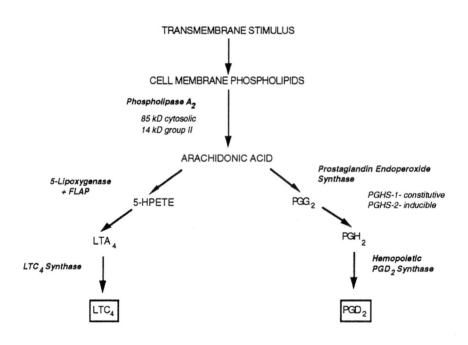

Fig. 1. Arachidonic acid metabolism in mast cells.

ENZYMES INVOLVED IN ARACHIDONIC ACID METABOLISM IN MAST CELLS

PLA_2

PLA_2 enzymes catalyze liberation of free fatty acids from the *sn*-2 position of glycerophospholipids. This reaction serves as one of the rate-limiting steps for biosynthesis of eicosanoids and of platelet-activating factor. To date, two classes of PLA_2s have been characterized in mammalian cells (22,23). There are 14-kDa secretory PLA_2s (sPLA_2s), subdivided into type I (pancreatic) and type II (non-pancreatic), and an 85-kDa cytosolic PLA_2 (cPLA_2). In contrast to the relatively restricted distribution of type I PLA_2 in pancreas, type II PLA_2 and cPLA_2 are distributed in a wide variety of cells and tissues, including mast cells; and their expression and functions are regulated independently by a number of transmembrane stimuli.

The rapid and fairly selective release of arachidonic acid from membrane phospholipids after cellular activation with various kinds of agonists suggests the role of cPLA_2, which is activated during the process of stimulus-coupled signal transduction. cPLA_2 hydrolyzes phospholipids bearing arachidonic acid much more efficiently that those bearing other fatty acids (24-27). It contains a region showing high homology with the calcium-dependent membrane-binding domain (CaLB domain) found in several proteins (26,27). The catalytic activity of cPLA_2 increases sharply with an increase in calcium concentration from submicromolar to micromolar, which corresponds to the range of change in cytosolic calcium concentration when cells are activated (24-27). This increase in activity is accompanied by CaLB domain-dependent translocation of the enzyme from the soluble to the membrane fraction (27). cPLA_2 contains a consensus phosphorylation site for mitogen-activated protein (MAP) kinase (26,27), which serves as a convergence point that integrates diverse signal transduction pathways (28). *In vitro* cPLA_2 activity is increased several fold via phosphorylation by MAP kinase (29,30). Although cPLA_2 phosphorylation *per se* is insufficient for arachidonic acid release *in vivo*, simultaneous increases of calcium and MAP-kinase-directed phosphorylation synergistically activate cPLA_2, leading to enhanced release of arachidonic acid (29,30). In a separate action, treatment of mast cells (21) or several cell lines (31-33) with particular cytokines stimulates an increase in gene expression of cPLA_2. The involvement of a certain G protein in the regulation of cPLA_2 activation has also been demonstrated (34). When BMMC are activated by FcεRI-crosslinking, cPLA_2 undergoes transient phosphorylation that parallels arachidonic acid release; and subsequently its expression is increased so that the cells release more arachidonic acid in response to a secondary stimulus that raises the cytoplasmic calcium concentration (35).

sPLA_2s hydrolyze phospholipid substrates to release fatty acids without specificity for arachidonic acid in the presence of millimolar concentrations of calcium. Inflammatory exudate contains type II PLA_2 (36,37). Injection of type II

PLA$_2$ into inflamed sites exacerbates the inflammation (38). Inflammatory cells, including mast cells, store the enzyme in secretory granules for release by exocytosis upon stimulation (39,40). Proinflammatory stimuli such as endotoxin or proinflammatory cytokines such as IL-1, IL-6, and tumor necrosis factor (TNF) α upregulate the gene expression and secretion of type II PLA$_2$ in a wide variety of cells, accompanied by increased production of eicosanoids (41-45). Type II PLA$_2$ is often detected as a cell surface-associated form through binding to heparan sulfate proteoglycan, which appears essential in order for this enzyme to exert its biological activity toward target cells (46-48). Although the involvement of type II PLA$_2$ in IgE-dependent eicosanoid generation in mast cells appears not so significant, it may participate in the regulation of degranulation (49,50).

PGHS   (Cyclooxygenase)

PGHS catalyzes two sequential reactions: a cyclooxygenase reaction in which arachidonic acid is converted to PGG$_2$ and a peroxidase reaction in which PGG$_2$ undergoes a two electron reduction to PGH$_2$. There are two PGHS isoforms, PGHS-1 and PGHS-2, each with a molecular mass of ~70 kDa (51). Within a species there is about 60% amino acid identity between these two isozymes (52-54). PGHS-2 contains an 18-amino acid insert near the C-terminus of the enzyme that is absent from PGHS-1, but all residues identified as essential for the catalytic activity of PGHS-1 are conserved in PGHS-2. Both isoforms are heme-containing integral membrane proteins that appear to exist as dimers and are located on the luminal side of the endoplasmic reticulum and/or nuclear envelope (55).

PGHS-1 is expressed constitutively in almost all tissues and cells, with generally minimal induction by cytokines (56-58). Apparently, cells use PGHS-1 to produce prostanoids needed to regulate "housekeeping activities" typically involving rapid responses to agonists, such as thrombogenic thromboxane A$_2$ generation by platelets, anti-thrombogenic prostacyclin production by vascular endothelial cells, cytoprotective prostanoid generation in the gastric mucosa, and renal blood flow-regulatory prostanoids production by the kidney. The PGHS-1 gene has a TATA-less promoter, a feature common to housekeeping genes (59).

PGHS-2 is induced rapidly and dramatically in response to proinflammatory cytokines, growth factors, lipopolysaccharide, phorbol esters, cAMP-elevating agents, and several G-protein-coupled agonists (52-54,60-65). Thus, induction of PGHS-2 is controlled transcriptionally by multiple signaling pathways, such as cAMP, protein kinase C, and tyrosine kinase pathways. PGHS-2 mRNA has multiple RNA instability sequences (AUUUA) in its 3'-untranslated region, suggesting significant regulation of the transcript by control of RNA degradation (52-54). PGHS-2 protein is also much less stable than is PGHS-1 (66). Dexamethasone can reduce PGHS-2 expression by suppressing PGHS-2 gene transcription and by reducing PGHS-2 mRNA stability (61-65). PGHS-2 apparently produces prostanoids that function during specific stages of cell differentiation or replication.

Non-steroidal anti-inflammatory drugs inhibit cyclooxygenase activity, thereby producing a variety of pharmacologic effects, including anti-pyretic, analgesic, anti-inflammatory, and anti-thrombogenic effects. Aspirin transfers its acetyl group from salicylate to a specific "active site" serine residue of PGHS-1 and PGHS-2, leading to irreversible inactivation of the enzymes (67,68). The beneficial effect of low-dose aspirin as an anti-thrombogenic agent results from its irreversible action on PGHS-1 present in platelets, which lack the necessary machinery for new protein synthesis. Indomethacin binds non-covalently and reversibly to both isoforms in a first phase, followed by a conformational change in the enzymes associated with tighter binding (69). Aspirin or indomethacin are more selective for PGHS-1 than PGHS-2, thereby causing peptic ulceration and impaired renal function as side effects (70). Recently, inhibitors relatively selective for PGHS-2 have been developed, such as NS-398 (71). These reagents have analgesic and anti-inflammatory activities with minimal gastric and renal toxicity (72).

PGD$_2$ Synthase

Two PGD$_2$ synthase enzymes have been described. A 28-kDa brain-specific enzyme that does not require glutathione (GSH) has been cloned and is a member of the lipocalin family of proteins, consisting of hydrophobic small molecule transporters (73). The other enzyme is 26-kDa hematopoietic PGD$_2$ synthase, initially identified in rat spleen and subsequently shown by immunochemical and biochemical criteria to exist in rat CTMC and in antigen-presenting cells (74,75). The hematopoietic enzyme depends on GSH for its activity, is localized to the cytosol, and possesses GSH S-transferase activity. The N-terminal amino acid sequence of rat hematopoietic PGD$_2$ synthase is similar to that of cytosolic GSH S-transferases (76). Its cDNA has not yet been cloned.

5-LO

5-LO catalyzes the metabolism of arachidonic acid to the unstable intermediate, 5S-hydroperoxyeicosatetraenoic acid, which is converted by the sequential action of the same enzyme to an epoxide, LTA$_4$. 5-LO is an 80-kDa cytosolic, or possibly nucleosolic metalloenzyme that translocates to the nuclear membrane on cell activation in a calcium-dependent manner (77-81). In subcellular assays, 5-LO requires calcium and ATP for its enzymatic activity. After mouse BMMC are stimulated with A23187, 5-LO associates irreversibly with the cell membranes and is permanently inactivated, whereas after IgE/antigen stimulation, 5-LO transiently associates with the membrane in accordance with a transient increase in intracellular calcium concentration and returns to the cytosol as an active enzyme (82). Whereas the promoter region of the 5-LO gene shares characteristics in common with the promoters of housekeeping genes, which are usually constitutively expressed in multiple tissues, 5-LO is expressed primarily in cells of myeloid or mast cell lineage (83,84).

The activity of 5-LO depends on an 18-kDa perinuclear protein, FLAP (85). MK-886, a drug that suppresses leukotriene biosynthesis in cells but does not inhibit 5-LO activity in cell lysates, is an inhibitor of FLAP. FLAP is likely central to the perinuclear presentation of released or translocated arachidonic acid to 5-LO (86).

LTC$_4$ Synthase

LTC$_4$ synthase, an integral microsomal membrane protein, conjugates LTA$_4$, an epoxide intermediate, with reduced GSH to form LTC$_4$. A cDNA encoding human LTC$_4$ synthase has recently been cloned from a KG-1 cell cDNA library (87). The nucleotide and deduced amino acid sequence have revealed a novel protein with a molecular mass of ~17 kDa, which shows no significant homology to GSH S-transferases but shows a 31% overall amino acid identity with FLAP. Moreover, LTC$_4$ synthase can be inhibited by the FLAP inhibitor, MK-886. Therefore, LTC$_4$ synthase is distinct from the known GSH-S-transferases, and its GSH-conjugating function represents a distinct integral membrane protein belonging to a newly recognized gene family, which also includes FLAP.

CYTOKINE PRIMING FOR INCREASED IGE-DEPENDENT PGD$_2$ GENERATION

We have examined the effect of KL and other mast cell-regulatory cytokines on the generation of PGD$_2$ and LTC$_4$ in BMMC in response to crosslinking of FcεRI. BMMC, developed in WEHI-3 conditioned medium as a source of IL-3, were cultured with KL alone or in combination with various accessory cytokines, sensitized with IgE, and stimulated with hapten-specific antigen. BMMC cultured with KL alone exhibited a 3-fold increase in PGD$_2$ generation; and the increase reached 6-8-fold when KL was combined with IL-3, IL-9, or IL-10, relative to BMMC maintained in IL-3 alone (21). The increased IgE-dependent PGD$_2$ generation was apparent after 1 day of culture and reached a maximum after 2 to 4 days. Other cytokines, including IL-1β, IL-6, TNF-α, IFN-γ, TGF-β1, and NGF, had no effect alone or in combination with KL, indicating that the accessory cytokines were selective. IgE-dependent LTC$_4$ synthesis increased less than 2-fold during BMMC culture with KL and was not influenced by the presence of accessory cytokines.

In order to identify the biochemical steps leading to increased PGD$_2$ synthesis in cytokine-treated BMMC, the changes in expression of the individual enzymes involved in the post-receptor metabolism of arachidonic acid to PGD$_2$ were assessed. Assays for mRNA expression by RNA blotting, for expressed protein by

SDS-PAGE/immunoblotting, and for activity of each enzyme revealed that KL stimulated the increased expression of the initial, the intermediate, and the terminal enzymes, namely $cPLA_2$, PGHS-1, and hematopoietic PGD_2 synthase (21).

Increased expression of $cPLA_2$ protein by BMMC was detectable after 10 h of culture with KL and reached a maximum at 2 days, coincident with a plateau for increased IgE-dependent generation of PGD_2 and LTC_4. There were minimal changes in $cPLA_2$ transcript, indicating post-transcriptional regulation of $cPLA_2$ expression. KL alone was sufficient for the increase in $cPLA_2$; and the accessory cytokines, IL-3, IL-9, and IL-10, did not enhance the effect of KL on $cPLA_2$.

The expression of PGHS-1 protein was increased 1 day after the start of the cell culture in the presence of KL, was near maximum by day 2, and plateaued at 4 to 7 days. Increased expression of PGHS-1 protein was preceded by increased expression of steady-state levels of PGHS-1 mRNA. Similar time-dependent changes in PGHS-1 protein were observed after treatment of the cells with KL + IL-3, KL + IL-9, and KL + IL-10. KL alone mediated increased expression of PGHS-1; and the accessory cytokines, IL-3, IL-9, and IL-10, each enhanced its expression further. In contrast, steady-state transcripts and protein for PGHS-2 were detected only during the initial 6 to 12 h of culture with KL + IL-10 and disappeared by 1 day, before cytokine priming for increased IgE-dependent PGD_2 generation occurred. These results indicate that the constitutive isoform of PGHS, with presumptive physiologic functions, rather than the inducible isoform, with putative pro-inflammatory functions, is the intermediate enzyme species responsible for cytokine priming of FcεRI-mediated prostanoid biosynthesis from endogenous arachidonic acid.

Hematopoietic PGD_2 synthase expression increased after 1 day of BMMC culture in KL, reached a maximum by 4 days, and was not affected by the addition of accessory cytokines. The time course of the increase in the enzyme expression was consistent with the change in the profile of IgE-dependent PGD_2 synthesis. The presence of GSH was necessary for PGD_2 synthase activity. Thus, hematopoietic PGD_2 synthase may be a further regulatory step in the priming of BMMC for increased IgE-dependent PGD_2 generation.

Thus, cytokine priming of BMMC for increased prostanoid synthesis by IgE/antigen is linked to increased expression of $cPLA_2$, PGHS-1, and PGD_2 synthase, but not PGHS-2 (Fig. 2). The optimal cytokine combination for induction of PGHS-1 involves accessory cytokines that do not elicit further induction of expression of $cPLA_2$ and PGD_2 synthase. Because the expression of 5-LO and FLAP was unchanged, the small increase in LTC_4 generation may be accounted for by the increased expression of $cPLA_2$, although the expression of the terminal enzyme in the 5-LO pathway, LTC_4 synthase, has not yet been examined (21). Nevertheless, the selective augmentation of PGD_2 generation relative to LTC_4 is compatible with the notion that KL leads to maturation of BMMC toward a CTMC-like phenotype (8,9).

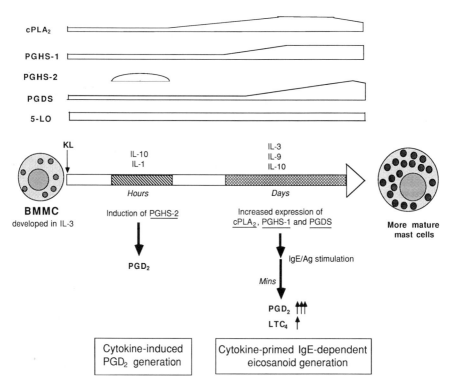

Fig. 2. Cytokine regulation of arachidonic acid metabolism in BMMC.

CYTOKINE-INDUCED PGD$_2$ GENERATION

When BMMC were cultured with KL in combination with IL-10 and/or IL-1β, PGHS-2 mRNA and protein were expressed transiently in a dose- and time-dependent fashion, accompanied by substantial release of PGD$_2$ into the culture medium, over 5 to 10 h (10). BMMC did not release PGD$_2$ appreciably in response to IL-3 alone during 10 h of culture. The capacity of each cytokine combination to elicit PGD$_2$ generation was KL + IL-10 + IL-1β >> KL + IL-10 = KL + IL-1β > KL alone. The cytokine-directed PGD$_2$ generation occurred during 2 to 10 h of culture and appeared to be related to the induction and magnitude of PGHS-2 protein as assessed by SDS-PAGE/immunoblotting. Induction of PGHS-2 mRNA expression by these cytokines preceded PGHS-2 protein expression. IL-1β appeared to enhance PGHS-2 protein expression not only transcriptionally but also translationally. PGHS-2 mRNA and protein were not induced when BMMC were cultured with IL-10 or IL-1β in the absence of KL, indicating that KL is essential for PGHS-2 expression. Other cytokines, including IL-3, IL-6, IL-9, TNF-α,

IFN-γ, TGF-$\beta 1$, and NGF, had no effect alone or in combination with KL. Accordingly, cytokines that did not induce PGHS-2 did not elicit cytokine-induced PGD$_2$ generation.

In contrast to the induction of PGHS-2, no cytokine combination changed the amount of PGHS-1 protein during the initial 10 h culture period. Thus, the kinetics of expression of PGHS-1 and PGHS-2 and their cytokine dependence suggest that cytokine-initiated PGD$_2$ generation is dependent upon PGHS-2. Furthermore, priming for increased IgE-dependent PGD$_2$ generation was not apparent until 12 h of culture, when PGHS-2 protein was no longer detectable and when increased expression of PGHS-1 could be detected. The association of PGHS-2 with cytokine-induced PGD$_2$ generation was further facilitated by the observations that dexamethasone, which reduces expression of PGHS-2 but not PGHS-1, and a PGHS-2-selective inhibitor, NS-398, inhibited cytokine-induced PGD$_2$ generation almost completely without affecting IgE-dependent PGD$_2$ generation. Thus, cytokine-induced direct PGD$_2$ generation is mediated by PGHS-2 irrespective of the presence of PGHS-1. Conversely, PGHS-2, even when abundantly expressed, does not prime cells for increased IgE-dependent PGD$_2$ generation, which is regulated by PGHS-1 (Fig. 2). Therefore, not only are the expression of the two PGHS isoforms regulated separately, but they can be coupled to different transmembrane stimuli in BMMC at a time when both are present and functional (10).

IL-10 appears to be a unique accessory cytokine that can contribute both to cytokine-induced PGD$_2$ generation and to cytokine priming for augmented IgE-dependent PGD$_2$ generation in combination with KL (10,21). Furthermore, even in the absence of KL, IL-10 can support priming for augmented IgE-dependent PGD$_2$ generation when IL-3 is supplied to maintain viability. Thus, BMMC cultured with IL-3 + IL-10 for 2 days and activated with IgE/antigen generated ~17 ng PGD$_2$/10[6] cells, whereas BMMC cultured in IL-3 alone generated ~4 ng PGD$_2$/10[6] cells. This effect can be accounted for by the observation that IL-10 or IL-3 + IL-10 increased PGHS-1 mRNA expression approximately 4-fold, followed by increased expression of PGHS-1 protein, relative to BMMC cultured in IL-3 alone, with no increase in expression of cPLA$_2$ or hematopoietic PGD$_2$ synthase. Neither IL-10 alone nor IL-3 + IL-10 induced PGHS-2 expression, and thereby did not elicit cytokine-directed PGD$_2$ generation.

REFERENCES

1. Stevens RL and Austen KF. *Immunol. Today* 1989; 10:381-86.
2. Lewis RA, Soter NA, Diamond PT, Austen KF, Oates JA and Roberts LJ. *J. Immunol.* 1982; 129:1627-31.
3. Heavey DJ, Ernst PB, Stevens RL, Befus AD Bienenstock J and Austen KF. *J. Immunol.* 1988; 140:1953-57.
4. Nakano T, Sonoda T, Hayashi C, et al. *J. Exp. Med.* 1985;162:1025-43.

5. Razin E, Mencia-Huerta JM., Stevens RL, et al. *J. Exp. Med.* 1983; 157:189-201.

6. Galli SJ, Zsebo KM and Geissler EN. *Adv. Immunology* 1994; 55:11-96.

7. Zsebo KM, Williams DA, Geissler EN, et al. *Cell* 1990; 63:213-24.

8. Tsai M, Takeishi T, Thompson H, et al. *Proc. Natl. Acad. Sci. USA* 1991; 88:6382-86.

9. Gurish M, Ghildyal N, McNeil HP, Austen KF, Gillis S and Stevens RL. *J. Exp. Med.* 1992; 175:1003-12.

10. Murakami M, Matsumoto R, Austen KF and Arm JP. *J. Biol. Chem.* 1994; 269:22269-75.

11. Lee FT, Yokota T, Otsuka T, et al. *Proc. Natl. Acad. Sci. USA* 1986; 83:2061-65.

12. Eklund KK, Ghildyal N, Austen KF and Stevens RL. *J. Immunol.* 1993;151: 4266-73.

13. Van Snick J, Goethals A, Renauld J-C, et al. *J. Exp. Med.* 1989;169:363-68.

14. Moore KW, Vieira P, Fiorentino DF, Trounstine ML, Khan TA and Mosmann TR. *Science* 1990; 248:1230-34.

15. Ghildyal N, McNeil HP, Gurish M, Austen KF and Stevens RL. *J. Biol. Chem.* 1992; 267:8473-77.

16. Ghildyal N, McNeil HP, Stechschulte S, et al. *J. Immunol.* 1992; 149:2123-29.

17. Ghildyal N, Friend D, Nicodemus CF, Austen KF and Stevens RL. *J. Immunol.* 1993; 151:3206-14.

18. Matsuda H, Kannan K, Ushio H, et al. *J. Exp. Med.* 1991; 174:7-14.

19. Mekori YA and Metcalfe DD. *J. Immunol.* 1994; 153:2194-2203.

20. Wong GHW, Clark-Lewis I, Hamilton JA and Schrader JW. *J. Immunol.* 1984; 133:2043-50.

21. Murakami M, Matsumoto R, Austen KF and Arm JP. submitted.

22. Kudo I, Murakami M, Hara S and Inoue K. *Biochim. Biophys. Acta* 1993; 117:217-31.

23. Dennis EA. *J. Biol. Chem.* 1994; 269:13057-60.

24. Takayama K, Kudo I, Kim D-K, Nagata K, Nozawa Y and Inoue K. *FEBS Lett.* 1991; 282:326-30.

25. Kim D-K, Kudo I and Inoue K. *Biochim. Biophys. Acta* 1991; 1083:80-88.

26. Sharp JD, White DL, Chiou XG, et al. *J. Biol. Chem.* 1991; 266:14850-53.

27. Clark JD, Lin L-L, Kriz RW, et al. *Cell* 1991; 65:1043-51.

28. Davis RJ. *J. Biol. Chem.* 1993; 268:14553-56.

29. Lin L-L, Lin AY and Knopf JL.*Proc. Natl. Acad. Sci. USA* 1992; 89:6147-51.

30. Lin L-L, Wartmann M, Lin AY, Knopf JL, Seth A and Davis RJ. *Cell* 1993; 72:269-78.

31. Lin L-L, Lin AY and DeWitt DL. *J. Biol. Chem.* 1992; 267:23451-54.

32. Hoeck WG, Ramesha CS, Chang DJ, Fan N and Heller RA. *Proc. Natl. Acad. Sci. USA* 1993; 90:4475-79.

33. Schalkwijk CC, de Vet E, Pfeilschifter J and van den Bosch H. *Eur. J. Biochem.* 1992; 210:169-76.
34. Winitz S, Gupta SK, Qian N-X, Heasley LE, Nemenoff RA and Johnson GL. *J. Biol. Chem.* 1994; 269:1889-95.
35. Nakatani Y, Murakami M, Kudo I and Inoue K. *J. Immunol.* 1994; 153:796-803.
36. Kramer RM, Hession C, Johansen B, et al.*J. Biol. Chem.* 1989; 264:5768-75.
37. Seilhamer JJ, Pruzanski W, Vadas P, et al. *J. Biol. Chem.* 1989; 64,5335-38.
38. Murakami M, Kudo I, Nakamura H, Yokoyama Y, Mori H and Inoue K. *FEBS Lett* 1990; 268:113-16.
39. Hayakawa M, Kudo I, Tomita S, Nojima S and Inoue K. *J. Biochem. (Tokyo):* 988; 96:785-92.
40. Murakami M, Kudo I, Suwa Y and Inoue K. *Eur. J. Biochem.* 1992; 209: 257-65.
41.Crowl RM, Stoller TJ, Conroy RR and Stoner CR. *J. Biol. Chem.* 1991; 266: 2647-51.
42. Nakano T, Ohara O, Teraoka H and Arita H. *FEBS Lett.* 1990; 261:171-74.
43. Schalkwijk C, Pfeilschifter T, Marki F and van den Bosch H. *J. Biol. Chem.* 1992; 267:8846-51.
44. Nakazato Y, Simonson MS, Herman WH, Konieczkowski M and Seder JR. *J. Biol. Chem.* 1991; 266:14119-27.
45. Pfeilschifter T, Schalkwijk C, Briner VA and van den Bosch H. *J. Clin. Invest.* 1993; 92, 2516-23.
46. Murakami M, Kudo I and Inoue K.*J. Biol. Chem.* 1993; 268:839-44.
47. Barbour SE and Dennis EA. *J. Biol. Chem.* 1993; 268, 21875-82.
48. Suga H, Murakami M, Kudo I and Inoue K. *Eur. J. Biochem.* 1993; 218: 807-13.
49. Murakami M, Kudo I, Suwa Y and Inoue K. *Eur. J. Biochem.* 1992; 209: 257-65.
50. Murakami M, Hara N, Kudo I and Inoue K. *J. Immunol.* 1993; 151:5675- 84.
51. Vane J. *Nature* 1994; 367:215-16.
52. Xie W, Chipman JG, Robertson DL, Erikson RL and Simmons DL. *Proc. Natl. Acad. Sci. USA* 1991; 88:2692-96.
53. Fletcher BS, Kujubu DA, Perrin DM and Herschman HR. *J. Biol. Chem.* 1992; 267:4338-44.
54. Jones DA, Carlton DP, McIntyre TM, Zimmerman GA and Prescott SM. *J. Biol. Chem.* 1993; 268:9049-54.
55. Otto JC and Smith WL. *J. Biol. Chem.* 1994; 269:19868-75.
56. DeWitt DL and Smith WL. *Proc. Natl. Acad. Sci. USA* 1988; 85:1412-16.
57. Merlie JP, Fagan D, Mudd J and Needleman P. *J . Biol. Chem.* 1988; 263: 3550-53.
58. Funk CD, Funk LB, Kennedy ME, Pong AS and Fitzgerald GA. *FASEB J.* 1991; 5:2304-12.
59. Kraemer SA, Meadde EA and DeWitt DL *Arch. Biochem. Biophys.* 1992;

293:391-400.

60. Pilbeam CC, Kawaguchi H, Hakeda Y, Voznesensky O, Alander CB and Raisz LG. *J. Biol. Chem.* 1993; 268:25643-49.

61. O'Banion MK, Winn VD and Young DA. *Proc. Natl. Acad. Sci. USA* 1992; 89:4888-92.

62. Hla T and Neilson K. *Proc. Natl. Acad. Sci. USA* 1992; 89:7384-88.

63. Pritchard Jr. KA, O'Banion MK, Miano JM, et al. *J. Biol. Chem.* 1994; 269: 8504-09.

64. Reddy ST and Herschman HR. *J. Biol. Chem.* 1994; 269:15473-80.

65. Kester M, Coroneos E, Thimas PJ and Dunn MJ. *J. Biol. Chem.* 1994; 269: 22574-80.

66. DeWitt DL and Meade EA. *Arch. Biochem. Biophys.* 1993; 306:94-102.

67. DeWitt DL, El-Harith EA, Kraemer SA, et al. *J. Biol. Chem.* 1990; 265:5192-98.

68. Lecomte M, Laneuville O, Ji C, DeWitt DL and Smith WL. *J. Biol. Chem.* 1994; 269:13207-15.

69. Walenga RW, Wall SF, Setty BN and Stuart MJ. *Prostaglandins* 1986; 31: 625-37.

70. Meade EA, Smith WL and DeWitt DL. *J. Biol. Chem.* 1993; 268:6610-14.

71. Futaki N, Yoshikawa K, Hamasaka Y, et al. *General Pharmacol.* 1993; 24:105-10.

72. Masferrer JL, Zweifel BS, Manning PT, et al. *Proc. Natl. Acad. Sci. USA* 1994; 91:3228-32.

73. Nagata A, Suzuki Y, Igarashi M, et al. *Proc. Natl. Acad. Sci. USA* 1991; 88: 4020-24.

74. Urade Y, Fujimoto N, Ujihara M and Hayaishi O. *J. Biol. Chem.* 1987; 262: 3820-25.

75. Urade Y, Ujihara M, Horiguchi Y, Ikai K and Hayaishi O. *J. Immunol.* 1989; 143:2982-89.

76. Urade Y, Ujihara M, Horiguchi Y, et al. *J. Biol. Chem.* 1990; 265:371-75.

77. Samuelsson B and Funk CD. *J. Biol. Chem.* 1989; 264:19469-72.

78. Dixon RAF, Jones RE, Diehl RE, Bennett CD, Kargman S and Rouzer CA. *Proc. Natl. Acad. Sci. USA* 1988; 5:416-20.

79. Rouzer CA, Rands E, Kargman S, Jones RE, Register RB and Dixon RAF. *J. Biol. Chem.* 1988; 263:10135-40.

80. Woods JW, Evans JE, Ethier D, et al. *J. Exp. Med.* 1993; 178:1935-46.

81. Brock TG, Paine III R and Peters-Golden M. *J. Biol. Chem.* 1994; 269: 22059-66.

82. Malaviya R, Malaviya R and Jakschik BA. *J. Biol. Chem.* 1993; 268:4939- 44.

83. Funk CD, Hoshino S, Matsumoto T, Radmark O and Samuelsson B. *Proc. Natl. Acad. Sci. USA* 1989; 86:2587-91.

84. Matsumoto T, Funk CD, Radmark O, Hoo J-O, Jornvall H and Samuelsson B. *Proc. Natl. Acad. Sci. USA* 1988; 85:26-3.

85. Dixon RAF, Diehl RE, Opas E, et al. *Nature* 1990; 343:282-84.

86. Mancini JA, Abramovitz M, Martha EC, et al. *FEBS Lett.* 1993; 318:277-81.
87. Lam BK, Penrose JF, Freeman GJ and Austen KF. *Proc. Natl. Acad. Sci. USA.* 1994; 91:7663-67.

*Biological and Molecular Aspects of Mast Cell
and Basophil Differentiation and Function,*
edited by Y. Kitamura, S. Yamamoto, S.J. Galli, and
M.W. Greaves. Raven Press, Ltd., New York © 1995.

4

EXPRESSION OF TH1 AND TH2 CYTOKINES THAT CONTROL MAST CELL GROWTH

Naoko Arai, Yoshiyuki Naito, Esteban S. Masuda, Hyun-Jun Lee*,
Risako Tsuruta*, Hideharu Endo, Takashi Yokota* and
Ken-ichi Arai*.

*DNAX Research Institute of Molecular & Cellular Biology, Department of
Cellular Biology, Palo Alto, CA, and *The Institute of Medical Science, The
University of Tokyo, Tokyo, Japan*

T. Mosmann first described subsets of Th cells according to profiles of cytokine activities and secreted proteins, elucidating the pathogenesis of allergic responses, i.e., joint involvement of IgE producing B cells, mast cells/basophils, and eosinophils (1, 2), (Fig. 1). Th2 cells secrete cytokines such as IL-3, IL-4, and IL-5 which induce allergic reactions by regulating growth and/or differentiation of effector cells, mast cells/basophils, and eosinophils, while Th1 cells secrete cytokines including IL-2 and IFNγ. Evidence for cross-regulation of Th subsets has been reported where cytokines such as IFN-γ, secreted by Th1 cells, inhibit responses by Th2 cells. Furthermore, production of IL-10 by Th2 cells may account for their ability to down-regulate inflammatory and Th1 or cell-mediated immune responses (3). Recent observations from several laboratories have suggested that both effector cells, Th1 and Th2, are derived from a common precursor cell rather than from precursors already committed to either differentiation pathway (4, 5). To develop toward Th1 or Th2 cells, the microenvironment at the time of antigen presentation to the early stage of Th cells (naive T cells) seems to be critical (6). Involvement of cytokines such as IL-4, IFN-γ, and IL-12 in the differentiation of Th cells from uncommitted T cells is especially important (7). Thus, cytokines such as IL-4, IFNγ, and IL12 act on an early stage of uncommitted T cells and seem to induce changes in signal transduction pathways and/or in transcription factors that result in Th1 or Th2 specific cytokine expression.

A signaling system which leads to production of cytokines

Antigen is presented to T cells in the form of peptide bound to major histocompatibility complex (MHC), and this process triggers a series of biochemical events that finally lead to cell proliferation and activate the effector function, secretion of lymphokines. This involves a cooperative interaction between the T cell receptor TCR/CD3 complex and the accessory molecules CD4/CD8 and CD28. By phosphorylating TCRζ, a src-related protein tyrosine kinase (PTK), p56[lck], initiates an activation cascade by enabling the receptor to recruit downstream molecules. Thus phosphorylation of TCRζ creates binding sites for the PTK ZAP-70 (8). Phosphorylated TCRζ has also been reported to

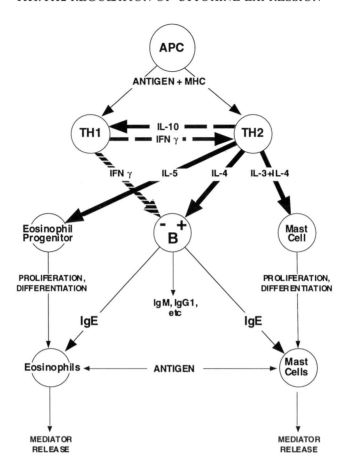

FIG. 1. Th1 and Th2 regulation of IgE responses
(courtesy of Dr. Robert Coffman)

bind to the intracellular SH2-domain-containing (SHC) adapter proteins (9). SHC proteins have been shown to link receptors to the activation of p21[ras]. Activation of p21[ras] by SHC is by means of the intermediate proteins Grb-2 and mSOS. mSOS is a guanine nucleotide-releasing protein, capable of exchanging GDP with GTP of p21[ras] (10). Vav is also reported to function as a guanine nucleotide releasing factor in the activation of Ras by T cell receptors (11). Thus ligation of the TCRζ/CD3 complex leads to the conversion of p21ras to an activated GTP-bound state. Kinase activity coupled to TCRζ/CD3-CD4 leads eventually to phosphorylation of the downstream target, PLCγ. Phosphorylated PLCγ then catalyzes the hydrolysis of phosphoinositol 4,5-diphosphate (IP3) and diacylglycerole (DAG), thereby mobilizing intracellular Ca^{2+} and stimulating protein kinase C (PKC). Thus TCR-mediated stimulation can be bypassed and effector function is elicited by activator of PKC, phorbol 12-myristate 13-acetate (PMA), and calcium ionophore.

In this way, Th clones, D10.G4.1 for Th2 and D1.1 for Th1, can be activated to secrete their respective cytokines with a combination of PMA and calcium ionophore by mimicking TCR mediated activation (12).

Activation of two signaling pathways, the PKC and calcium-dependent pathways, is strictly required, especially for expression of IL-2 and GM-CSF. Interestingly, addition of either PMA or calcium ionophore by itself induces cytokine production; i.e., expression of IL-3 and IL-4 is observed following activation of the calcium dependent pathway without the one dependent on PKC. On the other hand, IL-5 and IL-6 are secreted by activation of the PKC pathway only (12).

CsA is a widely utilized immunosuppressant and has been known to inhibit production of cytokines such as IL-2 by blocking the assembly of the transcription factor NFAT (13). A group of cytokines such as IL-2 and IL-4, whose expression was completely dependent on the activation of calcium pathway, was highly sensitive to CsA, while another group of cytokines, including IL-5 and IL-6, was relatively resistant to CsA inhibition due to partial dependency on calcium ionophore for their production. A similar observation was made even when different sets of Th clones were used (Naito, Y., unpublished observation). Therefore, we concluded that the signal requirements for induction of cytokines are unique to individual cytokines and do not discriminate between Th1 and Th 2.

PGE2, an arachidonic acid metabolite, is known as an immunosuppressant which elevates intracellular cAMP levels. Production of Th1 cytokines, such as IL-2, was inhibited by PGE2 as well as by agents which increase intracellular cAMP levels, including forskolin and cholera toxin (14, 15). This inhibition was observed when Th cells were stimulated by anti-CD3 or by PMA/calcium ionophore, although inhibition of cytokine production was less severe when cells were stimulated by PMA/calcium ionophore. On the other hand, production of Th2 cytokines was not inhibited by the addition of PGE2. Furthermore, IL-5 production was even upregulated by PGE2. This indicated that PGE2/cAMP discriminates Th1 from Th2 and that at least one target of cAMP action resides downstream of PKC and calcium.

Similarly, up- and down-regulations by cAMP were observed in EL-4, a mouse thymoma, which produced both Th1 and Th2 cytokines. Production of IL-2 was detected at both mRNA and protein levels when cells were treated by PMA without calcium. With the addition of Bt2cAMP in the culture medium, PMA-induced IL-2 expression was severely inhibited. On the other hand, IL-5 mRNA was detected only when cells were stimulated with PMA in the presence of Bt2cAMP. Either PMA or Bt2cAMP by itself, however, induces only a trace amount of IL-5 mRNA (16).

The target of Bt2cAMP inhibition on IL-2 promoter

In eukaryotic cells, sequences required for transcription initiation generally lie upstream of coding genes. The regulatory sequences consist of complex arrays of relatively short DNA sequence motifs. Each motif is a potential binding site for a specific protein, a transcription factor. To define a cis-acting DNA element, nuclease hypersensitive site mapping studies were routinely employed, followed by a fusion gene approach in which upstream sequences were fused to proper reporter genes such as chrolamphenicol acetyl transferase (CAT), luciferase, and β-galactosidase genes. After narrowing down regulatory sequences, DNA motifs required for regulation of cytokine gene expression were identified (Fig. 2). Then, DNA binding proteins which bind specifically to the motifs and probably account for the regulatory function of the motifs were detected using EMSA (electrophoretic mobility shift assay) and DNase I protection assays.

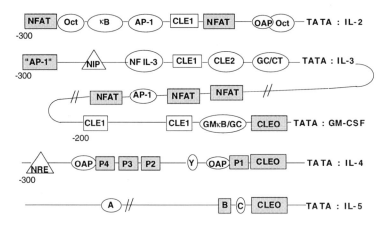

FIG. 2. Schematic representation of cis-acting DNA elements required for the expression of cytokines (IL-2, IL-3, GM-CSF, IL-4 and IL-5) by antigen stimulation through T cell receptor. Shadowed boxes indicate motifs with sequence similarity to CLE0 and NFAT binding sites.

We constructed fusion genes of CAT or luciferase with IL-2 and IL-5 genes carrying about 300 bp and 1200 bp of 5' upstream sequences, respectively. The IL-2 regulatory region has been well characterized and shown to contain NFAT, NF-κB, AP-1 and Oct motifs (17), (Fig. 2). As for IL-5, we recently identified three elements essential for IL-5 induction in addition to CLE0$_{IL-5}$ (conserved lymphokine element 0 for IL-5) (Fig. 2), (18). These constructs were transfected into EL4 cells by electroporation. As shown in Fig. 3, transcription from the IL-5 promoter was observed clearly only when both PMA and cAMP were present (Fig. 3, middle panel). In contrast, IL-2 expression observed with PMA stimulation was inhibited by the addition of 1 mM Bt2cAMP in the medium (Fig. 3, right panel). Furthermore, transfected protein kinase A (PKA) catalytic subunit substituted for cAMP effects (16). This indicated that negative and positive effects of cAMP on IL-2 and IL-5 transcription, respectively, were exerted through the activation of PKA. Transfection experiments in which IL-2 promoter carried mutations in binding sites for NFAT, NFκB, AP1, and Oct proteins indicated that multiple elements may contribute to negative responses to Bt2cAMP. Further analysis using constructs carrying multiple copies of NFAT site showed clear inhibition by Bt2cAMP when stimulated by PMA. In addition, treatment of EL-4 cells with Bt2cAMP enabled us to detect formation of NFκB homodimer (p50/p50) in place of heterodimer (p65/p50). This observation agrees with our previous observation using B21 cells, a human T cell clone (19). Interestingly, overexpression of NFATc abrogated the inhibitory action of Bt2cAMP. From these observations, we concluded that a major target for Bt2cAMP inhibition is NFAT, or NFκB, or both (20).

Cis-acting elements and their binding proteins which determine subset-specific expression

Why do Th1 cells specifically express cytokines for Th1 but not for Th2? To study differential expression of Th1 and Th2 cytokines, we first established an efficient procedure to introduce DNA into T cell clones. Earlier poor transfection efficiency had been a bottleneck for this study. Now we can transfect DNA into

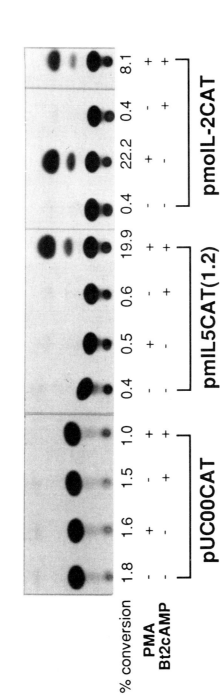

% conversion	1.8	1.6	1.5	1.0		0.4	0.5	0.6	19.9		0.4	22.2	0.4	8.1
PMA	-	+	-	+		-	+	-	+		-	+	-	+
Bt2cAMP	-	-	+	+		-	-	+	+		-	-	+	+
		pUC00CAT					pmIL5CAT(1.2)					pmoIL-2CAT		

FIG. 3.   Effect of Bt2cAMP on transfected IL-2 and IL-5 promoter sequences
fused to the chloramphenicol acetyl transferase (CAT) gene in EL4
cells. pUC00CAT is the vector alone and is included as a negative
control.

D10.G4.1 (Th2) and HDK1(Th1) cells with the efficiency of approximately0 10^{-3} by electroporation. We demonstrated that transfected IL-2 gene carrying 300 bp upstream regulatory sequences were expressed only in IL-2 producing cells, Th1, but not in non-producing cells, Th2. On the other hand, IL-5 construct having 1200 bp 5'-regulatory region was expressed only in Th2 cells. This indicates that transcription factor(s) interacting with the DNA element(s) located within 300 or 1200 bp upstream from transcription initiation site of IL-2 or IL-5 may determine subset specificity (Lee, H.-J., unpublished observation). Similarly, an IL-4 gene having 300 bp upstream region is sufficient to mediate transcriptional specificity in Th1 and Th2 subsets (21). Several reports, including ours, suggested that CLE0 for IL-4 and IL-5 and their binding proteins may explain mechanisms by which production of these cytokines could be differentially regulated in Th subsets (21, 22).

CLE0 (Conserved Lymphokine Element 0)

Our previous work on the regulation of mouse GM-CSF gene identified two essential elements within the region from position -95 to position +27 that mediate induction in response to phorbol ester and calcium ionophore (23). They are referred to as GM-kB/GC and CLE0 elements. Both GM-kB and CLE0 are targets for induction signals. Characterization of the factors recognizing $CLE0_{GM-CSF}$ revealed that one was similar to transcription factor AP1, and another had features similar to those of the nuclear factor of activated T cells (NFAT) (Fig. 4), (24).

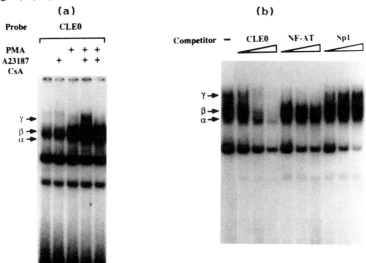

FIG. 4. NF-CLE0γ, whose binding is induced by PMA/calcium ionophore, is identical or related to NFAT. a, Nuclear extracts isolated by different stimulation conditions were incubated with labeled CLE0 oligonucleotides. b, Nuclear extracts from stimulated (PMA/calcium ionophore) were incubated with labeled CLE0 oligonucleotides with an excess of unlabeled competitor oligonucleotides at 0.5, 5, and 50 ng. α and β indicate binding by AP1 related molecules (Ref. 24).

Gene		Sequence
Consensus	(AP1 site)	TGA$_C^G$TCA
m,h GMCSF	(CLE0)	A<u>TTAATCAT</u> TTCC TCT
hIL2	(NFAT site)	<u>TGAAACAG</u>TTT TTCC TCC
mIL2	(NFAT site)	<u>TGAAACA</u>AATT TTCC TCC
hIL3	(AP1 site)	<u>TGAGTCAG</u>GC TTCC CCT
hIL4	(CLE0)	AAAC<u>TCA</u>TT TTCC CTC
mIL4	(CLE0/P$_0$)	AAAC<u>TCA</u>TT TTCC CTT
hIL4	(P)	GT<u>GAACGA</u>AAT TTCC AAT
hIL4	(PRE-I/P$_4$)	
mIL4	(P$_1$)	GT<u>GTAATA</u>AAATT TTCC AAT
mIL4	(P$_2$)	A<u>CAGGTA</u>AATT TTCC TGT
mIL4	(P$_3$)	GG<u>TGTTTC</u>ATT TTCC AAT
mIL4	(P$_4$)	TAT<u>GGTGTA</u>AT TTCC TAT
m,hIL5	(CLE0)	A<u>TTATTCA</u>T TTCC TCT
mIL5	(B)	CTG<u>AAACTCAG</u>GGT TTCC AGT
Consensus	(Ets site)	$^{AC}_{gt}$ TTCC $^{GCT}_{tGC}$

Table I. CLE0-like elements required for induction of transcription in T cells.

Consistent with this characterization, purified NFAT and purified AP1 bound the CLE0$_{GM-CSF}$ motif. Closer examination of CLE0$_{GM-CSF}$ revealed that its 5' half was similar to the AP1 binding site and that its 3' half had sequences similar to the NFAT binding site. As shown in Table I, this loose similarity can be extended to other cis-acting elements that are required for induction of cytokine expression. These elements are depicted schematically in Figure 2. As mentioned above, CLE0$_{IL-4}$ and CLE0$_{IL-5}$, which play a crucial role in conferring subset specificity, share homology with CLE0$_{GM-CSF}$. Similarly, the binding site for AP1 in the IL-3 promoter (25) and the binding site for NFP in the IL-4 promoter (26, 27), which are required for induction, also share homology wih CLE0 (28).

Is NFAT or a related protein involved in coordinate and/or differential expression of cytokine genes?

NFAT, which was first detected in the IL-2 system, is described as a heterotrimeric factor composed of a polypeptide of NFAT and of the heterodimer transcription factor AP1. The appearance of NFAT in the nuclear compartment requires both the activation of PKC and calcium mobilization. This translocation seems to depend on calcineurin, a protein phosphatase, and to be sensitive to the action of the immunosupressant CsA (17).

We purified NF-AT protein through affinity chromatography from nuclear extracts of human Jurkat cells stimulated with the combination of both PMA and calcium ionophore, A23187 (Fig. 5). We confirmed that the purified NF-AT bound to the CLE0 element and formed a NF-CLE0γ complex. One component of NF-AT with an apparent molecular mass of 120 kDa on SDS-polyacrylamide gel electrophoresis was purified to near homogeneity by MonoQ chromatography (29), (Fig. 5).

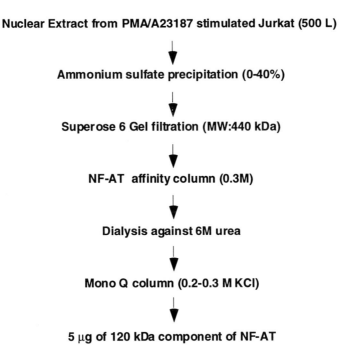

Nuclear Extract from PMA/A23187 stimulated Jurkat (500 L)

↓

Ammonium sulfate precipitation (0-40%)

↓

Superose 6 Gel filtration (MW:440 kDa)

↓

NF-AT affinity column (0.3M)

↓

Dialysis against 6M urea

↓

Mono Q column (0.2-0.3 M KCl)

↓

5 μg of 120 kDa component of NF-AT

FIG. 5.   Purification scheme of 120 kDa component of
the nuclear factor of activated T cells (NFAT).

We purified 120 kDa protein (5 μg) from activated Jurkat cell extract from
500 L of culture and digested it with LysC endopeptidase, and the resulting
peptides were sequenced. Isolation of cDNA fragments using PCR techniques
based on the amino acid sequence data was followed by cDNA library screening
to isolate full-length cDNA clones. We isolated three human clones, NFATc (30),
NFATp (31) and NFATx (32), a novel factor. We learned here that NFAT is
composed of a family of proteins. Subsequently, we found that they are encoded
by different genes and mapped on different chromosomes. There are three
distinct regions observed in the primary structure of NFAT proteins, i.e., an
amino-terminal region, a carboxyl-terminal region, and a middle region
containing the Rel-homology domain. The amino-terminal region of NFATx
showed more than 30% residues which were identical to analogous sequences
from NFATc and NFATp. The rel-homology domain is the most conserved
region within members of the NFAT family with more than 66% identical
residues. However, the carboxyl-terminal region showed no significant similarity
to the analogous sequences. Like other members of the NFAT family, DNA
binding activity of NFATx molecule was detected by Cos7-expressed NFATx. In
addition, transient transfection experiments in Jurkat cells as well as Cos7 cells
showed that IL-2 promoter activity increased 2-3 times when NFATx was
overexpressed, but only after activation by both PMA and calcium ionophore.
Although the different NFAT proteins are capable of binding the same NFAT-
binding site, their binding sequence specificity may not be identical. It remains to
be examined whether there are some preferences by a particular NFAT for
particular sites and whether there is a potential device for regulation at the
different cis-acting elements that bind NFAT.

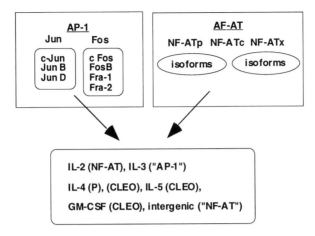

FIG. 6. Do combinations of members of the AP1 and the NFAT family of transcription factors determine which cytokines are expressed?

Furthermore, opportunities for additional regulation at NFAT-binding sites in various cytokine gene promoters are expanded when the diverse members of the AP1 family are considered (Fig.6). Further work is necessary to clarify the relative roles of the different components of NFAT in the regulation of expression of Th1 and Th2 cytokines. This knowledge ultimately will help us obtain a better understanding of the control of mast cell growth and function by cytokines.

ACKNOWLEDGMENTS

We thank R. Rodgers, G. Burget, and D. Wylie for their invaluable assistance in the preparation of this manuscript. DNAX Research Institute is supported by Schering-Plough Corporation.

REFERENCES

1. Mosmann, T.R., Cherwinski, H., Bond, M.W., Giedlin, M.A. and Coffman R.L. Two types of murine helper T cell clone, I. Definition according to profiles of lmphokine activities and secreted proteins. *J. Immunol* 1986; 136:2348.
2. Mosmann, T.R., and Coffman, R.L. Th1 and Th2 cells: Different patterns of lymphokine secretion lead to different functional properties. *Annu Rev Immunol* 1989;7:145.
3. Mosmann, T.R. and Moore, K.W. The role of IL-10 in cross-regulation of Th1 and Th2 responses. *Immunol Today* 1994; A49-A53.
4. Kamogawa, Y., Minasi, L., Carding, S.R., Bottomly, K. and Flavell, R.A. The relationship of IL-4- and IFN-γ-producing T cells studied by lineage ablation of IL-4 producing cells. *Cell* 1993;75:985-995.
5. Sad, S. and Mosmann, T.R. Single IL-2-secreting precursor CD4 T cell can develop into either Th1 or Th2 cytokine secretion phenotype. *J. Immunol* 1994; 153:3514-3521.
6. Le Gros, G., Ben-Sasson, S., Seder, R., Finkelman, F.D. and Paul, W.E. Generation of intereukin-4 (IL-4) producing cells *in vivo* and *in vitro*: IL-2 and IL-4 are required for *in vitro* generation of IL-4 producing cells. *J. Exp. Med.* 1990;172:921-929.
7. O'Garra, A. and Murphy, K. Role of cytokines in determine T-lymphocyte function. *Current Opinion in Immunology* 1994;6:458-466.
8. Chan, A.C., Irving, B., Fraser, J.D., and Weiss, A. The TCRζ chain associates with a tyrosine kinase and upon TCR stimulation associates with ZAP-70 M_r tyrosine phosphoprotein. *Proc Natl Acad Sci USA* 1991; 88:9166-9170.
9. Ravichandran, K.S., Lee, K.K., Songyang, Z., Cantley, L.C., Burn, P. and Burakoff, S.J. Interaction of Shc with the zeta chain of the T cell receptor upon T cell activation. *Science* 1993;262:902-905.
10. Rozakis-Adcock, M., Fernley, R., Wade, J.,Pawson, T. and Bowtell, D. The Sh2 and Sh3 domains of mammalian Grb2 couple the EGF receptor to the Ras activator mSos1. *Nature* 1993;363:83-85.
11. Gulbins, E., Coggeshall, K.M., Baier, G., Katzav, S., Burn, P. and Altman, A. Tyrosine kinase-stimulated guanine nucleotide exchange activity of Vav in T cell activation. *Science* 1993;260:822-825.
12. Arai, N., Naito, Y., Watanabe, M., Masuda, E.S., Yamaguchi-Iwai, Y., Tuboi, A., et. al., Activation of lymphokine genes in T cells: Role of cis-acting DNA elements that respond to T cell activation signals. *Pharmacol Ther (England)* 1992;55:303-308.
13. Flanagan, W.M., Corthesy, B., Bram, R.J. and Crabtree, G.R. Nuclear association of a T-cell transcription factor blocked by FK-506 and cyclosporin A. *Nature* 1991;352:803-807.
14. Betz, M., and Fox, B. Prostaglandin E2 inhibits production of Th1 lymphokines but not of Th2 lymphokines. *J. Immunol* 1991;146:108-113.
15. Novak, T.J., and Rothenberg, E.V. cAMP inhibits induction of interleukin-2 but not of interleukin-4 in T cells. *Proc Natl Acad Sci USA* 1991;87:9353-9357.
16. Lee, H-J., Koyano-Nakagawa, N., Naoto, Y. cAmP activates the IL-5 promoter synergistically with phorbol ester through the signaling pathway involving protein kinase A in mouse thymoma line EL-4. *J. Immunol* 1993; 151:6135-6142.

17. Crabtree, G.R. and Clipstone, N.A. Signal transmission between the plasma membrane and nucleus of T lymphocytes. *Annu Rev Boichem* 1994;63:1045-1083.

18. Lee, H.-J., Masuda, E.S., Arai, N., Arai, K. and Yokota, T. Characterization of the mouse interleukin 5 gene promoter: The role of an NF-AT relation factor. 1994, *Submitted.*

19. Watanabe, S., Yssel, H., Harada, Y. and Arai, K. Effects of prostaglandin E2 on T$_h$0-type human T cell clones: Modulation of functions of nuclear proteins involved in cytokine production. *Int. Immunol* 1994; 6:523-532.

20. Tsuruta, L., Lee, H.-J., Masuda, E.S., et. al. cAMP inhibits expression of the IL-2 gene through the NF-AT sequence and transfection of NF-AT cDNAs abrogates the sensitivity of EL-4 cells to cAMP. 1994, *Submitted.*

21. Bruhn, K.W., Nelms, K., Boulay, J.-L., Paul, W. and Leonard, M. Molecular dissection of the mouse interleukin-4 promoter. *Proc Natl Acad Sci USA* 1993; 90: 9707-9711.

22. Naora, H., van Leeuwen, B.H., Bourke, P.F. and Young, I. G. Functional role and signal-induced modulation of proteins recognizing the conserved TCATTT-containing promoter elements in the murine IL-5 and GM-CSF genes in T lymphocytes. *J. Immunol* 1994; 153: 3466-3475.

23. Miyatake, S., Shlomai, J., Arai, K. and Arai, N. Characterization of the mouse granulocyte-macrophage colony-stimulating factor (GM-CSF) gene promoter: Nuclear factors that interact with an element shared by three lymphokine genes--those for GM-CSF, interleukin-4 (IL-4) and IL-5. *Mol Cell Biol* 1991;11:5894-5901.

24. Masuda, E.S., Tokumitsu, H., Tsuboi, A., et al. The granulocyte-macrophage colony-stimulating factor promoter cis-acting element CLE0 mediates induction signals in T cells and is recognized by factors related to AP1 and NFAT. *Mol Cell Biol* 1993;13:7399-9407.

25. Shoemaker, S.G., Hromas, R. and Kaushanski, K. Transcriptional regulation of interleukin-3 gene expression in T lymphocytes. *Proc Natl Acad Sci USA* 1990;87:9650-9654.

26. Abe, E., de Waal Malefyt, R., Matsuda, I., Arai, K. and Arai, N. An 11-base pair DNA sequence motif apparently unique to the human inerleukin-4 gene confers responsiveness to T-cell activation signals. *Proc Natl Acad Sci USA* 1992;89:2864-2868.

27. Szabo, S.J., Gold, J.S., Murphy, T.L. and Murphy, K.M. Current understanding of IL-4 gene regulation in T cells. *Mol Cell Biol* 1993; 13:4793-4805.

28. Masuda, E.S., Naito, Y., Arai, K.and Arai, N. Expression of lymphokine genes in T cells. *The Immunologist* 1993;1:198-203.

29. Tokumitsu, H., Masuda, E.S., Tsuboi, A., Arai, K. and Arai, N. Purification of the 120 kDa component of the human nuclear factor of activated T cells (NF-AT): reconstitution of binding activity to the cis-acting element of the GM-CSF and IL-2 promoter with AP-1. *Biochem Biophys Res Commun* 1993;195:737-744

30. Northrop, J.P., Ho, S.N., Chan, L., et al. NF-AT components define a family of transcription factors targeted in T-cell activation. *Nature* 1994;369:497-502.

31. Jain, J., McCaffrey, P.G., Miner, Z., et al. The T-cell transcription factor NFATp is a substrate for calcineurin and interacts with Fos and Jun. *Nature* 1993;365:352-355.

32. Masuda, E.S., Naito, Y., Tokumitsu, H. et al. NFATx: A functional member of the NFAT family that is predominantly expressed in the thymus. 1994. *Submitted.*

Biological and Molecular Aspects of Mast Cell
and Basophil Differentiation and Function,
edited by Y. Kitamura, S. Yamamoto, S.J. Galli, and
M.W. Greaves. Raven Press, Ltd., New York © 1995.

5

Basophils as the Target and Source of Cytokines

Donald W. MacGlashan, Jr. and John T. Schroeder

Johns Hopkins University, Asthma and Allergy Center
5501 Hopkins Bayview Circle, Baltimore, Md. 21224

Today's view of allergic reactions, especially those involved in asthma, includes not only the release of mediators from mast cells but the recruitment of circulating leukocytes to the sites of allergen challenge to result in an allergic inflammatory process. There is specificity in this particular inflammatory reaction, it is dominated by eosinophils and lymphocytes as well as a reasonable number of basophils. The role of each of these cells in the maintenance of the allergic reaction is not altogether clear but in experimental models of the so-called late phase of the reaction (the cell recruitment phase), histamine appears to be derived from basophils that have entered the tissue. There are other chronic inflammatory reactions in which basophils appear to have an even greater presence. For example, in delayed-type hypersensitivity reactions (also classified as cutaneous basophil hypersensitivity), the basophil, normally less than 0.5% of circulating leukocytes, accounts for ≈15% of the leukocytes in the tissue reaction sites and appears prior to eosinophils which are the other dominant polymorphic leukocyte in these reactions [1]. Again, its pathophysiologic role is not clear. The basophil has many of the attributes of a leukocyte while also possessing the "machinery" for a mast cell-like response. It moves like a eosinophil or neutrophil and shares some receptors with these cell types but it also possesses a high affinity receptor for IgE antibody and relatively large granules containing histamine and other proteoglycans. Whether the signal transduction apparatus associated with IgE-mediated stimulation of these cells is identical to that of mast cells, is not yet entirely clear. However, it seems likely that some major features of this signalling pathway should be similar to mast cells and therefore the basophil can also be a surrogate for mast cells, thereby providing a more readily available source of cells for study of the IgE-mediated reaction in humans.

The paradigm shift that has occurred in our thinking about allergic reactions is two fold. The first is that this allergic inflammation may be partially responsible for the signs and symptoms of allergies and asthma and the second is that cytokines are primary mediators of these inflammatory reactions. While much of the evidence is not in place, it is unquestionably true that cytokines have a profound influence on cellular functions. In basophils, mediator release is markedly upregulated by treatment with interleukin-3 [2, 3]. Furthermore, following on the heels of reports that some murine mast cells line could synthesize cytokines, human basophils and mast cells have been shown to also secrete these substances [4-6]. For basophil studies, these two topics are currently intertwined because IL-4 release from these cells has most often been studied in the presence of IL-3 [7-9].

REGULATION OF BASOPHIL FUNCTION BY IL-3

During the last decade, a variety of studies have shown that basophil mediator release can be modified by cytokines. Cytokines which up-regulate basophil responses include IL-3 [2, 3], γ-IFN [3, 10] and stem cell factor [11], IL-5 [12, 13], and GM-CSF [2, 14] while weaker up-regulation occurs with IL-1 [15]. IL-8 has been reported to have inhibitory effects on chemokine or cytokine-induced release but the exact circumstances and reproducibility of the observations is less clear. There are a number of factors which induce outright release which have been called cytokines [16, 17] although from the standpoint of modulation alone, it is not clear that they fulfill this particular role. Of all these modifiers, IL-3 appears to be the most efficacious for up-regulating mediator release and can in fact induce release under appropriate conditions. IL-3 has been observed to enhance IgE-mediated LTC4 release from some donors over 100 fold [18]. On average, a 24 hour incubation with IL-3 causes a 10 fold increase in LTC4 release and a 3-fold enhancement of histamine release [3, 18]. As will be noted below, a similar treatment leads to a 8 fold increase in IL-4 release. These changes occur with an EC50 of ≈100 pmolar [3]. On the basis of these functions alone, these observations suggest that a good understanding of basophil function in an inflammatory reaction where cytokines are present requires a clear understanding of how and what IL-3 does to basophils. Not only are mediator release functions enhanced but other characteristics such as adherence are modified [19]. One might speculate that if a drug could be found that specifically inhibited the effects of IL-3 on basophil function (and that basophils had some role in these inflammatory reactions), by virtue of this effect alone, such a drug might profoundly alter the course of the inflammatory reaction. Discussing the search for the mechanism of the IL-3 effect is the topic of this section.

IL-3 is probably one of a few cytokines responsible for the development of basophils from more primitive cells. While other cytokines may play a role in the stable maturation of a basophil [20, 21], IL-3 certainly appears to have a central role. Given the current view that leukocytes are cells in the process of dying unless certain cytokines are present to prevent this apoptosis and that IL-3 promotes basophil differentiation, it is perhaps not surprising that IL-3 has such profound effects on basophil function. In order to understand the mechanism of the modulation it is useful to first note that IL-3 effects the response of basophils to all known secretagogues and it effects the secretion of all known mediators. These are important points because it is now quite clear that various basophil secretagogues employ different signal transduction pathways or that the secretion of different classes of mediators also employ different signal transduction pathways.

To expand on this point, a comparison of FMLP- and IgE-mediated secretion is useful. Anti-IgE antibody and FMLP result in similar secretion of both histamine and LTC4, however, other data indicates that the pathways to this similar mediator release must be quite different. For example, there is no correlation between the response of the basophil to FMLP and anti-IgE antibody [22]. The rates of secretion are markedly different; FMLP release is complete within 30-60 seconds while anti-IgE requires 10-15 minutes at a concentration optimal for release [22, 23]. Pharmacologic modulation shows clear dichotomies. The general kinase inhibitor, staurosporine, can completely inhibit IgE-mediated release while enhancing FMLP-induced release [24, 25]. Pertussis toxin inhibits FMLP while having no effect on IgE-mediated release [26]. Cyclosporine [27], cAMP active drugs [28], glucocorticosteroids [29] and okadaic acid [30] inhibit IgE-mediated release while having little or no effect on FMLP-induced release. There are other differences, including those at the level of known biochemical steps, but these serve to illustrate the apparently different signal transduction pathways used by these two secretagogues. The differences among all basophil secretagogues is even more extensive and yet IL-3 enhances the response to all stimuli. We have noted that the secretion of each of the 3 classes of mediators, histamine (granule contents), leukotrienes (early newly synthesized lipids), and IL-4 (late protein synthesis) probably involves certain early pathways that are distinct for each mediator and each mediator is independently regulated. IL-3 enhances the secretion of each type of mediator, regardless of the stimulus.

Therefore, IL-3 might alter something fundamentally required by all these different processes. However, the problem of finding this common point (if it is a common point) is made more difficult by the observation that the effects of IL-3 are two fold. A synthesis of the data from studies of both short and long incubations with IL-3 suggests that IL-3 has an immediate effect which differs in mechanism from the effects of a long preincubation. It is useful to note that enhancement of histamine or leukotriene release requires only 2-3 minutes, with the maximum initial effect clearly established by 15 minutes. This appears too short a time for significant protein synthesis to occur and experiments using cycloheximide show that protein synthesis is not required for enhancement to occur. When comparing short and long term incubations with IL-3, we make note of the following observations. Short pretreatments with IL-3 double histamine and leukotriene release following IgE-mediated stimulation. This initial level of enhancement is similar for pretreatment times ranging from 5 minutes to 2 hours. However, 24 hour pretreatments enhance LTC4 release 10 fold while histamine release is only marginally increased above the initial enhancement. In the above discussion of IL-4 release, we will note (see below) that short pretreatments with IL-3 had, on average, no effect on IL-4 release while enhancing histamine release. In contrast, 24 hour pretreatment led to an 8 fold increase in IL-4 release. Finally, we have noted that IL-3 can reverse the inhibition of histamine release by glucocorticosteroids. But if basophils are first treated with steroids for 24 hours and then for 15 minutes with IL-3, there is no reversal, only slight enhancement of the residual histamine release [3]. In contrast, including IL-3 in the cultures with steroid reverses the inhibition. Cells treated with IL-3 alone and cells treated with IL-3 and steroid show similar IgE-mediated histamine release. Taken together with some studies mentioned below, these observations indicate that there are two phases to the response to IL-3. This becomes more important when looking to the vast literature which exists describing some of the biochemistry of IL-3 on cell growth.

If IL-3 alters the response to all secretagogues and effects the release of all mediators, it should be altering some basic aspect of signal transduction, like the number of receptors. This later possibility seems unlikely since the receptors for all secretagogues would have to be increased in concert and in such a way that similar levels of enhancement would occur. Furthermore, it doesn't make sense for IgE-mediated release since both the number of high affinity IgE receptors and the IgE bound to the receptor would require up-regulation. The timing also seems too short (however, for other reasons, we have measured IgE-receptor densities ±IL-3 and did not find any changes in receptor density after 24 hr culture with IL-3). We have also considered the effect of IL-3 on ATP levels. All secretory reactions require energy and also involve phosphorylation of numerous components of the pathways. However, we have not found any effects of IL-3 on cellular ATP levels [31].

All physiologic stimuli studied to date cause an elevation in $[Ca^{++}]_i$ in basophils. These elevations are thought to be mandatory for secretion of each of the mediators although direct proof for this assertion is not available (indeed, there are now many reasons to consider this assertion false in the context of histamine release). Nevertheless, this also appeared to be a nexus for all secretagogues. We have examined the $[Ca^{++}]_i$ response which follows stimulation with anti-IgE antibody, FMLP, and C5a and in each case found enhancement of both histamine and leukotriene release in the absence of correlated changes to the $[Ca^{++}]_i$ response (in fact, is several preparations, some increase in the $[Ca^{++}]_i$ response did occur but because it wasn't consistent or correlated with enhance mediator release, it doesn't adequately explain the enhancement, see ref [31]). It should be noted that this is also an instance where the behavior following a short and long incubation differ. We have also found that the $[Ca^{++}]_i$ response following each of these stimuli is markedly enhanced following 24 hour pretreatment with IL-3 [32]. Clearly some change occurs during the longer incubation which does modify the early response to each stimulus. But just as clearly, this type of change doesn't account for the enhancement which follows short treatments with IL-3.

Many of the studies on how IL-3 alters cell growth and differentiation focus on observations that IL-3 changes the phosphorylation state of several cellular proteins and many studies focus on tyrosine phosphorylations as part of the signal transduction pathway proximal to the IL-3 receptor. For example, the JAK tyrosine kinases are now thought to be important in IL-3 receptor signaling. Some of the studies of IL-3 induced changes in cell growth have noted that the kinase inhibitor, staurosporine (which is reasonably selective for tyrosine kinases and PKC), often inhibits these early steps. However, staurosporine does not inhibit the ability of a 15 minute pretreatment with IL-3 to enhance C5a-induced leukotriene release (it should be noted that the absence of an effect on enhancement occurred in cells where the staurosporine was demonstrated to effect mediator release, i.e., staurosporine was demonstrably affecting some cellular process) [31, 33]. This is a surprising observation since it suggests that the acute effect of IL-3 does not involve any of the early reactions shown to occur in other cell systems where IL-3 effects growth. An even more surprising observation is that in a 24 hour pretreatment with IL-3, the presence of staurosporine also did not prevent the further enhancement of C5a-induced leukotriene release normally observed. Herbimycin, also a tyrosine kinase inhibitor (or down-regulator of SRC kinases), has similar inhibitory effects in the IL-3-dependent cell growth studies mentioned above. While we have not found that herbimycin can effect the IL-3-induced enhancement of LTC4 release, Krieger etal [33] has found that this tyrosine kinase inhibitor, as well as tyrphostin RG-50864 inhibit the IL-3 effect. These differences will need to be resolved.

In parallel with the studies on the effect of IL-3 on the calcium response, it was noted that IL-3 allows coupling of C5a stimulation to the generation of free arachidonic acid [31]. It should be pointed out that C5a, in the absence of IL-3 pretreatment, leads to no leukotriene release while inducing marked histamine release. A 5-15 pretreatment with IL-3 induces a qualitative change in behavior, under these conditions C5a can induce levels of LTC_4 release observed with FMLP or anti-IgE antibody [34]. The more recent studies showed that in the absence of IL-3, C5a induced little or no free arachidonic acid generation, presumably accounting for the absence of LTC4 release. IL-3 promoted the C5a-stimulated generation of free AA. In addition to this qualitative change in coupling, the rate of coupling was enhanced. In basophils stimulated with FMLP (also a fast stimulus like C5a), free AA generation and LTC4 release lag significantly behind histamine release, indeed, occurring after histamine release is complete [23]. IL-3 accelerates this coupling; following both C5a and FMLP, free AA generation occurs simultaneously with histamine release. These data suggest that IL-3 alters the coupling of the enzymes responsible for free AA generation. Unfortunately, the source of the free AA is not yet clear for basophils. Studies in other cell types, including rat or mouse mast cells, indicate that there are at least two major classes of phospholipase A2, the 14 kD and 85 kD varieties [35]. In some cells, both forms each account for some portion of the free AA generated [36]. The details for the generation of free AA in basophils are not yet clear. Preliminary studies in suggest that some of the free AA generated appears on the outside of the cell, a hallmark of the 14 kD-mediated process. On the other hand, this same free AA is not inhibited by a specific 14 kD inhibitor. In contrast, LTC4 release is inhibited by the same 14 kD inhibitor even while there is no effect on the free AA generated. The tentative conclusion is that there is a source of free AA which is normally completely metabolized to LTC4 (and therefore does not appear as measurable free AA) and this source is derived from the action of a 14 kD PLA2 on some phospholipid pool. It must be acknowledged that these are not the only ways that free AA can be generated, nor is this extremely dynamic process of AA generation and metabolism fully delineated. It might seem that altering free AA generation would only have a consequence to LTC_4 release (the only AA metabolite from basophils) but recent studies in rat mast cells have indicated that 14 kD PLA2 activity is mandatory for degranulation [37]. Numerous studies suggest a second messenger role for free AA: for example, free AA (and other unsaturated fatty acids) can alter the function of protein kinase C [38]. On the basis of several lines of evidence, we have suggested that PKC activation is the dominant pathway to degranulation in human basophils. Therefore, the fact that IL-3 can alter free AA generation might be important for both LTC_4 and histamine release (indirectly through PKC).

With the available information it is possible to speculate on how the various pieces of the puzzle fit together. A short term treatment leads to moderate enhancement of histamine and LTC4 release with little or no effect on IL-4 release. As free AA generation is altered by this treatment, it could directly effect LTC4 release and indirectly effect histamine release by affecting PKC activity or some other signal transduction pathway. The lack of an effect by IL-3 on the calcium response might explain the lack of effect on IL-4 release. However, following 24 hours treatment with IL-3, marked changes occur in the calcium response as well. At this point stimulation results in enhanced responses not only for histamine release, but the calcium-dependent metabolism of free AA by 5-lipoxygenase is also up-regulated even beyond the effect of having more available free AA. In addition, the enhanced calcium response then also augments the generation of IL-4 (see below). There are clearly many pieces of the story that have yet to be understood before this speculation finds a firm foundation. For example, acute IL-3 enhances PMA-induced histamine release. This is remarkable, in the context of the above statements, because the response to PMA may be a consequence of selective activation of the PKC-dependent pathway. Indeed, PMA induces no calcium response [24]. It might appear that this fits the scenerio since IL-3 alters free AA generation and free AA up-regulates PKC activity except for the fact that PMA induces no free AA generation in the presence of IL-3 (or its absence). Indeed, it suppresses even the very low resting levels of free AA. These experiments suggest that there are other effects of acute IL-3 but more work needs to be done.

IL-4 RELEASE FROM HUMAN BASOPHILS

Until several years ago, mediator release from mast cells and basophils was restricted to a study of either granule contents like histamine or newly synthesized lipid mediators like the leukotrienes. Even at this level, it was becoming apparent that the release of histamine could be dissociated from the release of leukotrienes. In pharmacologic studies, leukotriene release could be completely inhibited while histamine release was unaffected (although the reverse situation has not been found). Generally, this results from selective inhibition of the enzymes or steps just preceding the final metabolic steps of arachidonic acid conversion to leukotrienes. In addition to these pharmacologic maneuvers, some stimuli could be found to differentiate between these two pathways. For example, C5a could induce marked histamine release in the complete absence of measurable LTC4 release [23]. Likewise, phorbol esters like PMA could induce histamine release in the absence of LTC4 release [23]. Indeed, this stimulus can actively suppress LTC4 release while still promoting histamine release. These studies suggest that there is some independent regulation of different types of mediator release. After providing some background on IL-4 release from basophils, the discussion will return to this issue.

In 1989, Plaut, Wodnar-Filipowicz and others showed that murine mast cell lines could secrete a variety of cytokines following IgE-mediated stimulation [4, 5]. Similar studies have know shown this to be true for human mast cells or basophils [7-9]. In our studies, we have demonstrated both changes in IL-4 protein and its mRNA [9]. Typical studies of purified basophils still include a moderate number (10-20%) of contaminating lymphocytes and monocytes. Since IL-4 is a known cytokine product of T-cells, it is important to demonstrate that a stimulus like anti-IgE antibody does not first stimulate the basophil to secrete and then indirectly stimulate T-cells which might also be present. To exclude this possibility we examined IL-4 release under two conditions. The most critical studies compared IL-4 release from basophils from the same preparation at various levels of purification. A summary of the experiments where two purities of basophils were compared is shown in table 1. Both at the level of mRNA expression, with and without stimulation, and IL-4 protein secretion, the data indicated that basophils were the sole source of IL-4. In addition to this type of comparison, basophils were also purified to 99+% by positive selection on an anti-IgE coupled magnetic bead. While this type of experiment doesn't have an entirely appropriate negative control, it does show that very pure basophils produce similar levels of IL-4 protein. These studies provided convincing evidence that basophils can synthesize and secrete this cytokine. Indeed, it was found that the contaminants in these preparations do not secrete very much IL-4 even when stimulated with Con A and A23187. In particular, the kinetics of secretion from lymphocytes is quite different from basophils. We have observed that while IgE-mediated IL-4 release from basophils requires less than 4 hours ($T_{1/2}$ of 2 hours, with little or no release before 30 minutes). IL-4 release from lymphocytes requires 24 hours with little or no release at times less than 4 hours.

Table 1: Comparison of IL-4 protein secretion and mRNA expression in basophils at high and low purities

IL-4 protein	%purity	%HR	IL4R*	expected
stimulated	92±3	84±4	17.0±4	
stimulated	10±2	76±10	1.3±0.6	2.0
IL-4 mRNA	*purities (%)*	*band ratio***		*expected*
resting	91 vs 6	6.1±2.7		7.9
stimulated	91 vs 6	7.9±3.8		7.9

*   IL4R - IL-4 secretion, in pg/10^6 basophils
**   band ratio - ratio (expressed as %) of the optical densities of IL-4 PCR bands, (band density for lower purity basophils)/(band density for higher purity)

Several interesting observations resulted from these preliminary studies. While the pilot experiments used a short preincubation with IL-3 prior to stimulation, it was later found that this IL-3 was not necessary. With or without IL-3, basophils would secrete on average 30 pg/10^6 cells of IL-4 with a range of 10-70. There was no measurable spontaneous release of IL-4 and the addition of EGTA would stop its secretion. In addition, 1-2 μg/ml of cycloheximide also stopped secretion. Lysis of resting cells or cells post stimulation indicated that no IL-4 was cell associated. Taken together with the kinetic data, these observations indicate that IL-4 is newly synthesized.

The average of 30 pg/10^6 cells is low when compared to the studies by Brunner etal. [7]. However, we did make the observation that a long pretreatment, 18-24 hrs. did result in significant enhancement of IL-4 secretion. This was an interesting observation: a 15 minutes pretreatment with IL-3 would enhance histamine release by 100% while having no effect on IL-4 release (the data is mixed, clear by moderate enhancement in some cell preparations with clear but moderate inhibition of others). In contrast, a longer pretreatment enhanced the release of both mediators. After a long pretreatment with IL-4, IL-4 release averaged 190 pg/10^6 cells for a 6-10 fold increase above what is released in the absence of IL-3 pretreatment. This particular issue will be discussed in more detail below. The early basophils studies in laboratory relied on basophils that required approximately 24 hours to prepare. More recently, we have examined IL-4 release from basophils prepared by a simple two-step Percoll gradient (10-30% basophils). These cells are more responsive in general and IL-4 release remains associated with basophil stimulation and not the contaminating cells. Under these condition, IL-4 release averaged 190 pg/10^6 basophils (range 40-630). We also found no difference between atopic and non-atopic donors.

A more unexpected observation, and one which remains somewhat controversial, is that resting basophils expressed some mRNA for IL-4. Under conditions where the kinetics of mRNA expression could be observed, anti-IgE stimulation led to a ≈10 fold increase in the mRNA expression. However, these studies also made it clear that there was indeed a resting expression of IL-4 mRNA. While most of these studies were done using RT-PCR, which could easily expand a miniscule amount of IL-4 mRNA and give the appearance of significant resting expression, the relative expression in the context of stimulated cells removed some of this concern. In addition, we found that the resting expression in cells examined by competitive RT-PCR and by direct Northern blots supported the basic observation. Since this resting expression also was associated with the basophils and not the contaminant cells, it appears to be relevant to the basophil studies. It remains to be seen whether the basophils are experiencing a low level of stimulation due to their age or handling.

These studies also indicated that there was a loose correlation between the amount of histamine release and IL-4 secretion. But interestingly, a stimulus like goat polyclonal anti-IgE antibody led to some dissociation in the release of the two mediators. The basic observation is that the optimum concentration for IL-4 release occurs 5-10 fold lower than for histamine release. Indeed, at the optimum concentration for histamine release, IL-4 secretion has decreased to one-half the release observed at its optimum. Preliminary experiments with antigen indicate that this separation in the optimums does not occur as clearly. In fact the optimums following antigenic stimulation are not statistically different. This result may not be as strange as it appears and may in fact reveal something about the nature of signaling by different sized IgE/receptor aggregates. It has been known for some time that polyclonal anti-IgE is an unusual stimulus. It is the one IgE-mediated stimulus that can induce patching and capping of the receptor on basophils [39]. A synthesis of many lines of investigation suggests that the typically narrow dose response associated with polyclonal anti-IgE results from large aggregate formation on the supraoptimal side of the dose response curve [40]. Since release reactions are actually a dynamic process, a consequence of both activation and desensitization events, the rate at which these large aggregates form is important. At the optimum for histamine release, all that is important is that the large aggregates form slowly enough that they don't significantly interfere with the rate of histamine release (<30 minutes). However, since IL-4 release depends on functional crosslinks (see below), a slower accumulation of non-functional large aggregates during a 2-6 hr. time period using concentrations which are optimal for *histamine release* could actually result in poorer IL-4 release than lower concentrations of anti-IgE. Necessarily, the optimum for IL-4 release then occurs at lower concentrations of anti-IgE antibody.

This IL-4 story is particularly interesting for its implications to IgE-mediated signal transduction. In a typical IgE-mediated release reaction, the granule contents of the cell are rarely completely secreted. Indeed, release is often restricted to less than 50% of available histamine [18, 41]. At optimal levels of stimulation, a plot of the kinetics of histamine release shows a rapid release between 5 and 15 minutes after which the reaction reaches a plateau well below 100% release. Suboptimal stimulation (either side of the antigen dose response curve) leads to less release, further highlighting the fact that release appears to be down-regulated throughout the course of the reaction, leading to less than the maximal response. We have hypothesized that a natural process of desensitization regulates this reaction although only indirect proof is available for this hypothesis. Nevertheless, it is clear that histamine release is stopped within 15-30 minutes at a level less than maximum. IL-4 release occurs long after histamine release is complete. Apparently, those down-regulatory events which shut off histamine release had no impact on cytokine release. It appeared that two pathways were operating, one which led to degranulation and its specific control and another which led to cytokine release. In both cases, however, active crosslinks were required throughout either process. In an elegant series of experiments performed a decade ago, it was shown that histamine release initiated by a bivalent hapten like BPO_2 (bivalent penicillin) could be rapidly stopped by the addition of monovalent hapten (BPO-lysine) [42]. Adding BPO-lysine at any time during the release reaction would stop histamine release as effectively as adding EGTA. A similar observation was made for the secretion of cytokines from murine mast cell lines or BMMC [43]. We have recently observed the same behavior for IL-4 release from basophils sensitized with penicillin-specific IgE and challenged with a low valency BPO(7)-HSA conjugate. Adding BPO-lysine to the reaction after histamine release was complete but prior to significant IL-4 releaase halted further IL-4 release. This is shown by harvesting some cellular supernatants at the time of BPO-lysine addition and comparing these to supernatants harvesting much later. Therefore, the secretion of IL-4, throughout its time course, requires the maintenance of whatever early signals are generated by aggregating IgE receptors (and despite the fact that the same receptors no longer signal histamine release). A similar experiment using EGTA to stop the reaction showed the same result, with the implication that extracellular calcium was required throughout secretion as well. A synthesis of these various results suggests that desensitization events are specific for the mediator examined. Each type of mediator, preformed granule contents, newly synthesized acute lipid mediators and newly synthesized proteins, has its own release pattern, although histamine and LTC4 are certainly grouped in the same early time period.

Recent studies in basophils suggest that the cytosolic calcium ($[Ca^{++}]_i$) response is one early signal that is required for secretion. As noted above, we speculate that ongoing histamine release is regulated by a coincident process of desensitization. Several years ago we hypothesized that this desensitization process down-regulated the cytosolic calcium response which follows IgE-mediated stimulation. The assumption was that a $[Ca^{++}]_i$ response was required for the maintenance of histamine release. However, we have subsequently found that the cytosolic calcium response is only slowly down-regulated following its initial rise during the time period preceding histamine release [44]. In other words, the slight decay towards resting levels that was observed could not account for the cessation of histamine release. As it turns out another early signal, the activation of PKC, does show a more appropriate decay [45]. But this leaves a mystery as to the role of the prolonged elevation in $[Ca^{++}]_i$ and why in a desensitization style experiment, the $[Ca^{++}]_i$ response also decays so slowly. The explanation may lie with its role in maintaining the IL-4 release reaction. Possibly, the prolonged elevation in $[Ca^{++}]_i$ supports the events leading to IL-4 secretion. An examination of IL-4 release kinetics shows that even this process is eventually stopped, presumably by some internal regulatory events. A desensitization style experiment provides a complement to these studies. In this type of experiment, anti-IgE is added to cells in the absence of external calcium, for various periods of time, after which calcium is added to start the full reaction. In this type of protocol, subsequent histamine release approaches zero with a decay constant of $\approx$15 minutes. Both the $[Ca^{++}]_i$ response and the decay of IL-4 release have decay constants on the order of 30-45 minutes. These results suggest a relationship between control of the $[Ca^{++}]_i$ response and IL-4 release.

If elevations in cytosolic calcium are a requirement for IL-4 release, then stimuli like FMLP or C5a should cause histamine release in the absence of IL-4 release because the calcium signals decay rapidly with these stimuli. A synthesis of our results with both highly purified basophils and basophils enriched by the single 2-step Percoll gradient indicate that both stimuli only poorly induce IL-4 secretion. Indeed, in the majority of basophil preparations, no release is observed. But it is equally clear that some IL-4 release does occur in some preparations (this release also appears is highly purified cells). There is a 7 fold difference in cytosolic calcium decay rates for IgE-mediated and FMLP-mediated stimulation, 894±162 vs 132±20 secs respectively. In preparations which do release IL-4 in response to FMLP, there is 8 fold less IL-4 release when secretion is normalized to the amount of histamine release (this is done to account for initial differences in signal strength). These two results are therefore consistent with the necessity for a sustained calcium response. Furthermore, if the distribution of cytosolic calcium decay rates in FMLP-stimulated basophils is plotted for 68 different preparations of basophils analyzed for calcium changes, it can be seen that only a minority of preparations show long enough decay rates to mimic the IgE-mediated response. This result is also consistent with the observation that only a minority of basophil preparations show IL-4 release in response to FMLP. Further studies are required to prove that these associations are meaningful.

These studies of IL-4 secretion are really in the preliminary stages. It is clear that basophils can secrete IL-4 in response to IgE-mediated stimulation and that secretion is a consequence of newly synthesized protein. While IL-4 can be secreted in the absence of an up-regulator like IL-3, IL-3 markedly enhances its secretion. The biological significance of this capability is entirely unclear. It remains to be seen if basophils secrete other cytokines and whether there are independent pathways of regulation for this particular function of the basophil.

REFERENCES

1.   Dvorak HF, Mihm MC Jr. Basophilic leukocytes in allergic contact dermatitis. *J. Exp. Med.* 1972;135:235-254.

2. Hirai K, Morita Y, Misaki Y, et al. Modulation of human basophil histamine release by hematopoetic growth factors. *J. Immunol.* 1988;141:3957-3961.
3. Schleimer RP, Derse CP, Friedman B, et al. Regulation of human basophil mediator release by cytokines. I. Interaction with antiinflammatory steroids. *J Immunol* 1989;143(4):1310-7.
4. Plaut M, Pierce JH, Watson CJ, Hanley HJ, Nordan RP, Paul WE. Mast cell lines produce lymphokines in response to cross-linkage of Fc epsilon RI or to calcium ionophores. *Nature* 1989;339(6219):64-7.
5. Wodnar-Filipowicz A, Heusser CH, Moroni C. Production of the heamopoetic growth factors GM-CSF and interleukin-3 by mast cells in response to IgE receptor-mediated activation. *Nature* 1989;339:150.
6. Young JD, Liu CC, Butler G, Cohn ZA, Galli SJ. Identification, purification, and characterization of a mast cell-associated cytolytic factor related to tumor necrosis factor. *Proc Natl Acad Sci USA* 1987; 84(24):9175-9.
7. Brunner T, Heusser CH, Dahinden CA. Human peripheral blood basophils primed by interleukin-3 (IL-3) produce IL-4 in response to immunoglobulin E receptor stimulation. *J. Exp. Med.* 1993;177:605-611.
8. MacGlashan DW, Kagey-Sobotka A, White J, Huang SK, Lichtenstein LM. Human basophils generate IL4. *Clin. Res.* 1993;41:137A.
9. MacGlashan J D.W., White JM, Huang SK, Ono SJ, Schroeder J, Lichtenstein LM. Secretion of interleukin-4 from human basophils: The relationship between IL-4 mRNA and protein in resting and stimulated basophils. *J. Immunol.* 1994;152:3006-3016.
10. Hernandez AM, Hooks JJ, Ida S, Siraganian RP, Notkins AL. Interferon-induced enhancement of IgE-mediated histamine release from human basophils requires RNA synthesis. *J Immunol* 1979;122(4):1601-3.
11. Columbo M, Horowitz EM, Botana LM, et al. The effect of recombinant human c-lit receptor ligand, rhSCF, on mediator release from human skin mast cells. *Int. Arch. All. App. Immunol.* 1993; in press.
12. Bischoff SC, Brunner T, De WAL, Dahinden CA. Interleukin 5 modifies histamine release and leukotriene generation by human basophils in response to diverse agonists. *J Exp Med* 1990;172(6):1577-82.
13. Hirai K, Yamaguchi M, Misaki Y, et al. Enhancement of human basophil histamine release by interleukin 5. *J Exp Med* 1990;172(5):1525-8.
14. Bischoff SC, de Weck AL, Dahinden CA. Interleukin 3 and granulocyte/macrophage-colony-stimulating factor render human basophils responsive to low concentrations of complement component C3a. *Proc Natl Acad Sci USA* 1990;87(17):6813-7.
15. Massey WA, Randall TC, Kagey SA, et al. Recombinant human IL-1 alpha and -1 beta potentiate IgE-mediated histamine release from human basophils. *J Immunol* 1989;143(6):1875-80.
16. MacDonald SM, Lichtenstein LM, Proud D, et al. Studies of IgE-dependent histamine releasing factors: heterogeneity of IgE. *J Immunol* 1987;139(2):506-12.
17. Kuna P, Reddigari SR, Schall TJ, Rucinski D, Sadick M, Kaplan AP. Characterization of the human basophil response to cytokines, growth factors, and histamine releasing factors of the intercrine/chemokine family. *J Immunol* 1993;150(5):1932-43.
18. Nguyen KL, Gillis S, MacGlashan DW Jr. A comparative study of releasing and nonreleasing human basophils: nonreleasing basophils lack an

early component of the signal transduction pathway that follows IgE cross-linking. *J Allergy Clin Immunol* 1990;85(6):1020-9.

19. Bochner BS, Mckelvey AA, Sterbinsky SA, et al. Il-3 Augments Adhesiveness for Endothelium and Cd11B Expression in Human Basophils But Not Neutrophils. J Immunol 1990;145(6):1832-1837.

20. Donahue RE, Seehra J, Metzger M. IL-3 and GM-CSF act synergistically in stimulating hemotopoiesis in primates. *Science* 1988;241:1820-1823.

21. Sillaber C, Geissler K, Scherrer R, et al. Type beta transforming growth factors promote interleukin-3 (IL-3)-dependent differentiation of human basophils but inhibit IL-3-dependent differentiation of human eosinophils. *Blood* 1992;80(3):634-41.

22. Siraganian RP, Hook WA. Mechanism of histamine release by formyl methionine-containing peptides. *J Immunol* 1977;119(6):2078-83.

23. Warner JA, Peters SP, Lichtenstein LM, et al. Differential release of mediators from human basophils: differences in arachidonic acid metabolism following activation by unrelated stimuli. *J Leukoc Biol* 1989; 45(6):558-71.

24. Warner JA, MacGlashan DW Jr. Signal transduction events in human basophils - A comparative study of the role of protein kinase-C in basophils activated by anti-IgE antibody and formyl-methionyl-leucyl-phenylalanine. *J Immunol* 1990;145(6):1897-1905.

25. Knol EF, Koenderman L, Mul FPJ, Verhoeven AJ, Roos D. Differential activation of human basophils by anti-IgE and formyl-methionyl-leucyl-phenylalanine. Indications for protein kinase C-dependent and -independent activation pathways. *Eur. J. Immunol.* 1991;21:881-5.

26. Warner JA, Yancey KB, MacGlashan DW Jr. The effect of pertussis toxin on mediator release from human basophils. *J Immunol* 1987;139(1):161-5.

27. Cirillo R, Triggiani M, Siri L, et al. Cyclosporin A rapidly inhibits mediator release from human basophils presumably by interacting with cyclophilin. *J Immunol* 1990;144(10):3891-7.

28. Botana LM, MacGlashan DW Jr. Effect of cAMP-elevating drugs on stimulus-induced cytosolic calcium changes in human basophils. *J. Leuk. Biol.* 1994;in press.

29. Schleimer RP, MacGlashan DW Jr., Gillespie E, Lichtenstein LM. Inhibition of basophil histamine release by anti-inflammatory steroids. II. Studies on the mechanism of action. *J. Immunol.* 1982;129:1632-1636.

30. Botana LM, MacGlashan DW Jr. Effect of okadaic acid on human basophil secretion. *Biocheml Pharm* 1993;45:2311-2315.

31. MacGlashan JDW, Hubbard WC. Interleukin-3 alters free arachidonic acid generation in C5a-stimulated human basophils. *J. Immunol.* 1993;151:6358-6369.

32. MacGlashan DW Jr., Warner JA. Stimulus-dependent leukotriene release from human basophils: A comparative study of C5a and Fmet-leu-phe. *J Leuk. Biology* 1991;49:29-40.

33. Krieger M, von-Tscharnar V, Dahinden CA. Signal transduction for interleukin-3 dependent leukotriene synthesis in normal human basophils: opposing role of tyrosine kinase and protein kinase. *Eur. J. Immunol.* 1992;22:2907-2913.

34. Kurimoto Y, de Weck AL, Dahinden CA. Interleukin 3-dependent mediator release in basophils triggered by C5a. *J Exp Med* 1989;170(2):467-79.

35. Murakami M, Kadu I, Umeda M, et al. Detection of three distinct phospholipse A2 in cultured mast cells. *J. Biochem.* 1992;111:175.

36. Fonteh AN, Chilton FH. Mobilization of different arachidonate pools and their roles in the generation of leukotrienes and free arachidonic acid during immunologic activation of mast cells. *J. Immunol.* 1993;150:563-570.

37. Murakami M, Kudo I, Suwa Y, Inoue K. Release of 14-kDa group II phospholipase A2 from activated mast cells and its possible involvement in the regulation of the degranulation process. *Eur. J. Biochem.* 1992;209:257-265.

38. Shinomura T, Asaoka Y, Oka M, Yoshida K, Nishizuka Y. Synergistic action of diacylglycerol and unsaturated fatty acid for protein kinase C activation: its possible implications. *Proc Natl Acad Sci USA* 1991; 88(12):5149-53.

39. Becker KE, Ishizaka T, Metzger H, Ishizaka K, Grimley PM. Surface IgE on human basophils during histamine release. *J Exp Med* 1973;138(2):394-409.

40. MacGlashan DW Jr., Mogowski M, Lichtenstein LM. Studies of antigen binding on human basophils. II. Continued expression of antigen-specific IgE during antigen-induced desensitization. *J Immunol* 1983;130(5):2337-42.

41. Knol EF, Mul FP, Kuijpers TW, Verhoeven AJ, Roos D. Intracellular events in anti-IgE nonreleasing human basophils. *J. All. Clin. Immunol.* 1992;90:92-103.

42. Sobotka AK, Dembo M, Goldstein B, Lichtenstein LM. Antigen-specific desensitization of human basophils. *J Immunol* 1979;122(2):511-7.

43. Paul WE, Seder RA, Plaut M. Lymphokine and cytokine production by FcεRI positive cells. *Adv. in Immunol.* 1993;53:1-29.

44. MacGlashan DW Jr. Single cell analysis of free cytosolic calcium changes in human lung mast cells: II. The relationship between desensitization and the cellular regulation of calcium changes. *Mol. Immunol.* 1991;28(6):585-597.

45. Warner JA, MacGlashan DW Jr. Protein kinase C (PKC) changes in human basophils. IgE-mediated activation is accompanied by an increase in total PKC activity. *J Immunol* 1989;142(5):1669-77.

Biological and Molecular Aspects of Mast Cell and Basophil Differentiation and Function, edited by Y. Kitamura, S. Yamamoto, S.J. Galli, and M.W. Greaves. Raven Press, Ltd., New York © 1995.

6

Cytokine-Mediated Signal Transduction in Mast Cells

J.W. Schrader, M.J. Welham, K.B. Leslie, and V. Duronio

The Biomedical Research Centre and the Department of Medicine, The University of British Columbia, Vancouver, BC, Canada, V6T 1Z3

The physiology and pathology of the mast cell are regulated by a series of cytokines. These cytokines coordinate the generation of mast cells by stimulating the proliferation and differentiation of mast cell precursors, but also act on mature mast cells, stimulating their proliferation and survival, and modulating effector functions, e.g. mediator release. The list of cytokines that affect mast cells is still growing and includes interleukin-3 (IL-3), interleukin-4 (IL-4), interleukin-9 (IL-9), and interleukin-10 (IL-10), Steel (or Stem-Cell) factor (SLF), and interferon α/β, and γ.

Mast cells have played an important role in the identification and characterization of new cytokines. The first instance was that of IL-3. The capacity of IL-3 to support the generation of homogenous populations of mast cells from murine bone-marrow (and other tissues) (41, 45, 46) and the dependence of these mast cells on IL-3 for their survival and growth formed the basis of an assay used to identify and purify IL-3 (10, 43). IL-9 was another cytokine that was first recognized as a co-stimulating factor, which enhanced the mitogenic response of IL-3 dependent bone-marrow mast cells to IL-3 (25), an action also shared with IL-4 (6) and IL-10 (49). Several of the groups that reported the initial molecular characterization of SLF used as an assay stimulation of proliferation of bone-marrow-derived or peritoneal mast cells (1, 32, 61). Murine IL-3-dependent mast cells were also one of the cells in which the capacity of interferon-γ to upregulate the expression of Class II major histocompatibility complex antigens was first recognized (63).

Two cytokines, IL-3 and SLF, are particularly important in stimulating the generation of mast cells from precursors, and administration of either IL-3 (44) or SLF (51) to animals, including primates, can result in marked mastocytosis. Both IL-3 and SLF also affect mature mast cells. One important effect is to maintain their viability. There are no detectable levels of IL-3 present in normal mice (43), and *in vitro* generated IL-3-dependent mast cells die rapidly if injected into the skin (13). Likewise, experiments on mice treated with SLF have shown that when the administration of SLF to mice is halted, the mast cells rapidly disappear (51).

IL-3 and SLF also regulate other functions. As noted, IL-3 antagonizes the action of interferon-γ in upregulating the expression of class II histocompatibility antigens on mast cells (62). SLF activates murine mast cells (60) and IL-3 and SLF enhance mediator-release from basophils (21, 24, 29) or mast cells (2).

IL-3, SLF and IL-4 also influence the differentiation of mast cells, each having distinct effects. In the mouse, IL-3 generates populations of mast cells which closely resemble the mucosal or thymus-dependent subpopulation of mast cells that have been extensively characterized in rodents (11, 42, 43). In contrast, SLF supports the generation of both mucosal and mast cells and bone-marrow mast cells that have more of the characteristics of connective tissue mast cells (51). New information on the regulation of genes encoding proteins characteristic of mast-cells, e.g. proteases (Stevens, ibid) is providing insights into how different cytokines e.g. IL-3 and SLF differentially regulate the promoters of different genes and thus exert distinct effects on mast cell differentiation. Such analyses should provide clues to differences in the transcription factors that are activated by triggering of the respective receptors and thus to the molecular basis of the characterization effects of these cytokines on mast cell differentiation. Because of the diversity of cytokines that affect mast cells and the variety of molecular markers that are available, mast cells should provide an excellent model system for gathering basic information on how different cytokines exert distinctive effects on cellular differentiation.

COMPLEXITY OF CYTOKINE SIGNALS

Mast cells have already provided important information on interactions between cytokines. This is an important topic because, *in vivo*, cells are always influenced by multiple cytokines, and these can interact in both positive and negative ways. One level of interaction influences the control of growth. For example, IL-3 and IL-4 show strong synergistic activity in stimulating the growth of murine peritoneal mast cells, either alone having no effect on growth (22, 52). IL-4 is unable to promote continued growth of IL-3 dependent bone marrow derived mast cells, only temporarily prolonging their *in vitro* survival (5). However, IL-4 synergizes strongly with SLF in promoting growth of these cells (J. Wieler and J. Schrader, unpublished data).

A second level of interaction lies in control of differentiation. In the case of the negative effect of IL-3 on the induction in mast cells of class II major histocompatibility complex antigens by IFN-γ (62), there is already a clue to the molecular mechanism in analysis of the inhibitory effect of IL-3 on the induction by IFNγ of FcγRI genes in monocytes. Thus IL-3 induces tyrosine phosphorylation of a transcription factor that competes for binding to a sequence in the promoter of the FcγRI gene with the transcription factor activated by interferon-γ (27).

Models of the signal transduction mechanisms triggered by cytokines in mast cells must take into account this variety of biological observations. One question is how different cytokines, utilizing quite different types of receptors, exert both common effects, such as stimulating or co-stimulating mast-cell growth or blocking apoptosis, as well as cytokine-specific effects, such as regulating a particular mast-cell protease gene. *In vitro* observations of synergy or antagonism point to interactions between signal transduction pathways triggered by different cytokines. Another complication is that none of the cytokines discussed is specific for mast cells. Some, like IL-3, are restricted in their actions to other derivatives of the pluripotential hemopoietic stem cell (42, 43). Others, like IL-4, not only regulate hemopoietic cells, and in particular the immune system, but also affect endothelial cells and fibroblasts. SLF has an important role not only in the development and physiology of pluripotential hemopoietic stem cell erythrocytes and mast cells, but is also involved during embryogenesis in the migration of germ cells, the precursors of melanocytes and certain neurons in the brain. The actions of a cytokine on a mast cell, may thus depend not only on the characteristics of the relevant receptor, but also on the presence or levels in that cell-type of components of signal transduction paths such as kinases or phosphatases or transcription factors.

CYTOKINE RECEPTORS ON MAST CELLS

Tyrosine Kinase Receptors

This discussion will focus on signal transduction by receptors of two major families. One family, exemplified by the receptor for SLF, the protein c-*kit*, is characterized by an intracellular tail that has intrinsic activity as a protein tyrosine-kinase. This enzymatic activity is conferred by two domains that, characteristically for this family, are separated by an intervening sequence of amino acids. The extracellular part of the receptor is characteristically made up of a series of immunoglobulin-like domains. Other members of the family are the receptors for CSF-1 (c-fms) and for the flk-2 or flt3 ligands (flk-2 or flt3). The ligands for these receptors, e.g. CSF-1, SLF, and FlK-2-ligand are also closely related. X-ray crystallographic analysis of CSF-1 indicates that perhaps surprisingly, these ligands have the same basic three-dimensional structure as the cytokines (IL-2, IL-4, GM-CSF, etc.), that bind to the second quite distinct family of receptors described below. Interestingly, the receptors for structurally unrelated cytokines, platelet-derived growth factor and the fibroblast growth factors are quite similar in their general extracellular and intracellular characteristics to c-kit, c-fms, and flt3. The ligands for these receptors exist as dimers and ligand-induced dimerization or oligomerization of the receptor subunits is thought to be instrumental in activating the enzymatic activity of these receptors.

Superfamily of Hemopoietin Receptors

The second family of cytokine receptors is a novel one only recognized in the past five years. It is now known to include the receptors for a wide range of cytokines - interleukins 2, 3, 4, 5, 6, 7, 9, 11, 12, 13, 15, granulocyte-macrophage colony stimulating factor (GM-CSF), granulocyte CSF, erythropoietin, ciliary neurotrophic factor, oncostatin-M, mpl-ligand and leukemia inhibitory factor (LIF), as well as of the conventional hormones, growth hormone and prolactin. Receptors of the hemopoietin-receptor family are typically made up of homodimers, hetero-dimers or hetero-trimers of subunits, all of which are members of the family (reviewed in 30). In contrast to the tyrosine-kinase receptors, none of these subunits has any intrinsic enzymatic activity. A common subunit structure, exemplified by the receptor for IL-3, is of a smaller α-chain that binds ligand with low-affinity and a larger β chain that, when complexed with the ligand and α-chain, generates a high affinity binding site (16, 30). Signal transduction is triggered by apposition of these subunits, which in a complex manner results in activation of a number of cytoplasmic kinases and phosphatases (Reviewed in 30).

TYROSINE PHOSPHORYLATION INDUCED BY SLF, IL-3, and IL-4

As expected from the structure of c-kit, where there is clear structural evidence of an intracellular tyrosine kinase domain, stimulation of mast cells with SLF activates kinase activity (32, 38, 58). The receptor itself is rapidly phosphorylated on tyrosine, presumably through trans-phosphorylation following ligand-induced dimerization (38). However, stimulation of IL-3 dependent mast cells with SLF also results in the rapid phosphorylation on tyrosine of numerous proteins, initially characterized in terms of their mobility on SDS-PAGE (58). In some instances, e.g. that of the MAP-kinases erk-1 and erk-2, it seems clear that these proteins are not direct substrates of c-kit. In the case of other tyrosine-phosphorylated proteins, it has yet to be established whether c-kit phosphorylates them directly or via activation of other tyrosine kinases. We started our investigation of cytokine-activated signal transduction in mast cells (58) by asking which of these tyrosine phosphorylation events were peculiar to the action of SLF, and which might reflect the engagement of common signal transduction paths like growth or apoptosis. We therefore compared the pattern of proteins that were tyrosine phosphorylated in mast cells in response to SLF with those tyrosine phosphorylated in response to IL-3 and IL-4, both of which acted via the receptors of the hemopoietin-receptor superfamily.

Although the IL-3 receptor lacks intrinsic tyrosine kinase activity, there was evidence that IL-3 stimulated the phosphorylation on tyrosine of a range of proteins (15, 31). We took populations of IL-3 dependent bone-marrow derived murine mast cells and compared the patterns of tyrosine phosphorylation induced by IL-3 with that induced by SLF (58). One or two-dimensional SDS-PAGE revealed both similarities and differences; clearly some of the tyrosine-phosphorylated proteins were common to IL-3 and SLF-stimulated cells, while others were peculiar to one or the other (Table 1). The common substrates included two proteins with Mr 42K and 44K, and one of about Mr 55K. SLF, but not IL-3, induced tyrosine phosphorylation of c-kit. Likewise, IL-3, but not SLF, induced tyrosine phosphorylation of a 135-150K band that was shown to correspond to the β chain of the IL-3 receptor (15). Following IL-3 treatment the Mr of the IL-3 receptor β chain rapidly changed from 120K to 135-150K, due mainly to additional phosphorylation on Ser or Threonine residues (15).

TABLE 1.   **Some of the Major Substrates of Kinase Activity Stimulated by IL-3, IL-4 and SLF in Mast Cells.**

Stimulus	Substrates		
	Mr (K)	Identity	Functional Role
SLF only	150	c-kit	SLF receptor
	77	?	?
IL-4 only	170	IRS-1 like	associates with PI-3 kinase.
IL-3 only	135-150	β chain IL-3 receptor	subunit of IL-3 receptor
	90	?	?
	70	?	?
SLF, IL-3	p50, p55	Shc	adaptor molecule; involved in activation of p21ras.
SLF, IL-3	p44	erk-1 (MAP kinases)	ser/thr kinase.
	p42	erk-2	

Cytokines and MAP Kinases.
The 42K and 44K bands were shown by enzymological and immunological techniques and two-dimensional gel electrophoresis to correspond to two serine-threonine kinases, erk-2 and erk-1, earlier characterized as MAP-kinases (55). These enzymes were known to be activated in response to a broad range of hormones and extra-cellular signals (3, 33, 48). We showed that coincident with tyrosine-phosphorylation of these enzymes, IL-3 and SLF stimulated the enzymatic activity of MAP kinases (55). Tyrosine-phosphorylation of these enzymes is known to increase their enzymatic activity, and is now known to be mediated by an enzyme, MEK, which is in turn activated by a serine-threonine kinase, raf-1 (3, 48).

Interestingly, unlike IL-3 or SLF, IL-4 failed to induce either tyrosine phosphorylation of p42 and p44 or stimulation of MAP-kinase activity. This was interesting, first because at least in certain factor-dependent myeloid or lymphoid lines, IL-4 was mitogenic and stimulated continuous growth (56). This suggested that in these lines IL-4 activated a novel path that complemented the MAP kinase path characteristic of all growth factors except IL-4 (56) and h-thyrotropin (26). Second, the failure of IL-4 to activate MAP-kinases correlated with the observation that it also failed to activate another intracellular event usually associated with stimulation of cellular growth, namely activation of p21[ras] (18, 40).

CYTOKINES AND ACTIVATION OF p21[ras]

The ras family of proteins are highly conserved small G-proteins that are associated with the transduction of signals from the cell-surface in a wide range of organisms including yeast, Dyctostelium and C. elegans. The importance of ras in regulation of mammalian cellular growth is highlighted by the fact that activating mutations of ras are found in 25-30% of all human cancers. Both IL-3 (18, 40) and SLF (18) induce activation of p21[ras], resembling in this other cytokines like GM-CSF, IL-2, erythropoietin (18) and IL-6. Strikingly, however, IL-4 failed to activate p21[ras] in factor dependent cells (18, 40) or T lymphocytes and bone-marrow derived mast cells (56). The activation of p21[ras] by both SLF, acting via the tyrosine-kinase receptor c-kit, and IL-3 acting through a hemopoietin-superfamily receptor were inhibited by inhibitors of tyrosine kinases (18). In contrast, inhibitors of protein-kinase C, which contributes to activation of p21[ras] via the antigen-receptors of T lymphocytes (14), had no effect on activation of p21[ras] induction by SLF and IL-3 (18).

Regulation of p21[ras]
The mechanisms whereby tyrosine kinases activated p21[ras] were long unclear. PDGF induced tyrosine phosphorylation of p120 GAP, a protein that tends to keep p21[ras] in its inactive state by enhancing the intrinsic GTPase activity of p21[ras], thereby favoring hydrolysis of p21[ras] bound GTP to GDP and inactivation of the p21[ras] (49) Neither IL-3 or SLF, however, induced tyrosine phosphorylation of p120 GAP (18). A clue to the role of IL-3- and SLF-induced tyrosine phosphorylation in activation of p21[ras] came from comparison of the

patterns of tyrosine phosphorylation induced by IL-4 (which failed to activate p21^{ras}) and IL-3 and SLF (which did).

Aside from the p42 and p44 identified as erk-1 and erk-2 and now known to be downstream of p21^{ras}, IL-3 and SLF, but not IL-4 induced tyrosine phosphorylation of a protein of Mr 50 and 55K. All the other cytokines that activated p21^{ras} - IL-2, erythropoietin, IL-5, GM-CSF, and CSF-1 - also induced tyrosine phosphorylation of this protein, which was a major substrate of cytokine-activated tyrosine kinase activity (17, 58). IL-4 failed to induce tyrosine phosphorylation of the 50 and 55K protein in all cell types investigated.

Effects of Cytokines on Shc

A protein termed Shc was known to associate with the activated EGF receptor and undergo tyrosine-phosphorylation. The Shc proteins had been characterized as a series of isoforms of Mr 46K, 52K, and 66K (35). The Shc protein had an SH-2 domain that mediated its binding to a phosphorylated tyrosine on the receptor and when tyrosine phosphorylated itself, was in turn recognized by the SH-2 domain of another linker protein termed grb2. The grb2 protein was the mammalian homologue of the product of the sem-5 locus of C. elegans, and genetic studies had shown that the sem-5 product functioned upstream of ras and downstream of a tyrosine-kinase receptor (28, 34, 47). Moreover, overexpression of Shc resulted in cellular transformation, consistent with the idea that Shc functioned upstream of grb2 and ras (35).

Therefore we performed experiments on mast cells stimulated with SLF, IL-3 or IL-4, using anti-Shc antibodies to identify Shc. These studies demonstrated that the p 50, p55 proteins that were tyrosine phosphorylated in response to SLF and IL-3 but not IL-4 were indeed Shc (54). Moreover, when mast cells were stimulated with IL-3, the tyrosine phosphorylated Shc was bound grb2 (54). These experiments showed for the first time that the ability of a growth factor to induce tyrosine phosphorylation of Shc correlated with its capacity to activate p21^{ras}.

FIGURE 1.   **Hemopoietins and Activation of p21^{ras}**

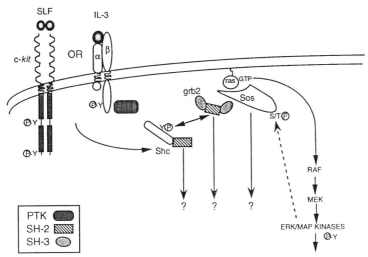

Cytokines and Sos1

Genetic studies in Drosophila had indicated that a cytoplasmic protein termed son-of-seven-less (Sos) functioned upstream of ras and downstream of a cell-surface receptor (sevenless) with tyrosine-kinase activity (37). This protein was shown to have activity as a guanine-nucleotide exchange factor that stimulated the exchange by ras molecules of GDP for GTP, thus putting the ras into its active conformation. Bowtell et al (4) had cloned a mammalian homologue of SOS, mSos1, and several groups showed that mSos1 was constitutively bound to grb2 (6, 19, 39). Buday and Downard reported that stimulation of Rat-1 fibroblasts with EGF resulted in translocation of mSos1 from the cytosol to the membrane (6). Based on this observation, they proposed a model that explained how activation of tyrosine-kinase-receptors resulted in activation of ras. Auto-phosphorylation of the activated receptor created a binding site for the SH-2 domain of grb2. When cytoplasmic grb2 associated with the cytoplasmic domain of the receptor, it brought with it to the cell-membrane the constitutively associated mSos1. It was this receptor-mediated relocation of mSos1 to the membrane that was postulated to bring mSos1 into close proximity with the membrane-associated ras. Association of mSos1 with ras then stimulated ras to exchange GDP for GTP. This model was made more attractive by lack of any evidence that growth factors stimulated any increase in the nucleotide exchange activity of mSos1.

Our observations on signal transduction in mast cells (54) indicate that cytokines that interact with receptors in the hemopoietin-receptor superfamily, also induce changes in mSos1. Treatment of mast cells with IL-3, as well as SLF, induced a change in the mobility on SDS-PAGE of mSos1. However, the kinetics of this change were delayed relative to activation of $p21^{ras}$ and reached a peak only 20-30 min after stimulation (54). Moreover, whereas previously we had shown that a specific inhibitor of protein kinase-C had no effect on activation of $p21^{ras}$ by IL-3 and SLF (18), this inhibitor partially blocked the shift in Mr of mSos1 induced by IL-3 and SLF (54). Thus in these two respects, the change in Mr of SOS-1 did not correlate precisely with activation of ras. However, in contrast to results with IL-3 and SLF, treatment of mast cells with IL-4 failed to induce this change in the Mr of mSos1 (54), an observation that correlated with the failure of IL-4 to induce tyrosine phosphorylation of Shc and activation of $p21^{ras}$.

Together these observations suggest that the change in Mr of SOS-1 did not precede and initiate the activation of $p21^{ras}$, but rather was a consequence of and was dependent upon $p21^{ras}$ activation. The decrease in mobility on SDS-PAGE of mSos1 induced by stimulation of fibroblasts with EDGF is due to phosphorylation on ser/thr residues (39). The m-SOS-1 sequence includes a number of potential sites for phosphorylation by MAP-kinases, and our data are consistent with the notion that mSos1 is phosphorylated on ser/thr by MAP-kinase. The functional significance of this modification of mSos1 is unknown; it may represent a down-regulatory mechanism or alternately activate other paths.

The model of Buday and Downward that has gained wide currency would predict that cytokines that activated ras would do so by initiating translocation of mSos1 from the cytoplasm to the cell membrane via the association of the linker or adapter molecules Shc and grb2 with a cell-surface receptor-associated complex.

The results of our experiments on the stimulation of mast cells with IL-3 and SLF, however, do not support this simple model. We were unable to detect significant biochemical translocation of mSos1 to the membrane after stimulation of mast cells with either SLF or IL-3. All of the modified mSos1 was detected in the cytosolic faction of the cell. Moreover, IL-3 and SLF also failed to stimulate translocation of Shc to the membrane. A very small fraction of Shc or grb2 was constitutively associated with the membrane and stimulation with SLF and IL-3 resulted in its tyrosine phosphorylation. Nevertheless, the vast majority of the tyrosine phosphorylated Shc - which bound grb2 - was detected in the cytosolic fraction (54).

We believe that these experiments based upon primary cultures of normal mast cells expressing physiological numbers of receptors are likely to provide a more accurate picture of the mechanisms activating ras than the experiments reported by Buday and Downward (6). Thus while it still seems likely that the tyrosine phosphorylation of receptors and receptor-associated molecules that are stimulated by cytokine-binding result in the association of Shc-grb2 mSos1 complexes with the receptor complex, these interactions are probably very transient. Importantly, the bulk of these complexes are found in the cytoplasm, and the possibility that they have novel functions in this site needs further investigation. Our results are not peculiar to mast cells, as we obtained similar results using EGF and Rat-1 cells.

INTERLEUKIN-4: A SPECIAL CASE

The failure of IL-4 to induce tyrosine phosphorylation of Shc and to activate the p21ras - MAP-kinase pathway is only one of the distinctive functions of IL-4 mediated signalling. IL-4 also induces tyrosine phosphorylation of a distinctive cytoplasmic protein of Mr 170 which we termed p170 and which Pierce and colleagues termed 4PS.(53). This occurs in mast cells, T and B lymphocytes, and myeloid cells. When tyrosine-phosphorylated, PI-3 associates strongly with the p85 subunit of PI-3 kinase, an enzyme which is activated by IL-4, as well as IL-3 and SLF (20). The p170/4PS protein is a similar size to IRS-1, which is heavily phosphorylated on tyrosine when non-hemopoietic cells are stimulated with insulin (59). In hemopoietic cells, however, insulin stimulates tyrosine phosphorylation of p170/4PS (unpublished data and 53). In appropriate cells IL-13 also stimulates growth phosphorylation of p170/4PS (M. Welham and J. Schrader, unpublished data). Tyrosine phosphorylation of p170/4PS does not seem to be critical for the growth-promoting effects of IL-4, as tyrosine phosphorylation of p170/4PS does not occur in response to IL-4 in a T cell line CT4.S that grows continuously in IL-4 (54).

OTHER ASPECTS OF SIGNAL TRANSDUCTION

Mast cells provided an interesting example of another type of interaction between different cytokines. We found that IL-3, but not IL-4, was able to downregulate c-*kit* mRNA and protein in mast. This may represent a mechanism which released mast cells (and hemopoietic stem cells) from SLF-bearing stromal cells. It is also another example of how that IL-3 and IL-4 exert distinct effects on mast cells (57).

We have not discussed here the molecular structure of the IL-3 and IL-4 receptors, as this topic is covered by Dr. Arai and colleagues. Nor have we discussed the nature of the non-receptor tyrosine-kinase(s) and phosphatases that are activated by cytokine action. This is a complex subject with good evidence for the activation of both JAK family and *src*-family tyrosine kinases and for the involvement of tyrosine-phosphatases.

There is evidence that IL-3 and IL-4, probably via activation of members of the JAK family, induce tyrosine phosphorylation of members of the STAT family of latent cytoplasmic transcription factors. Tyrosine phosphorylation results in the formation of homo- or hetero-dimers and translocation to the nucleus, where they bind to specific sequences and regulate the promotion of genes. As noted, the antagonism between IL-3 and IFN-γ observed in experiments on mast cells, may result from competition between STAT transcription factors activated by IL-3 and IFN-γ. Like other growth factors, IL-3, IL-4, and SLF also induce expression of transcription factor genes like c-myc, c-jun, and c-fos.

FIGURE 2   **Signal Transduction by Hemopoietins**

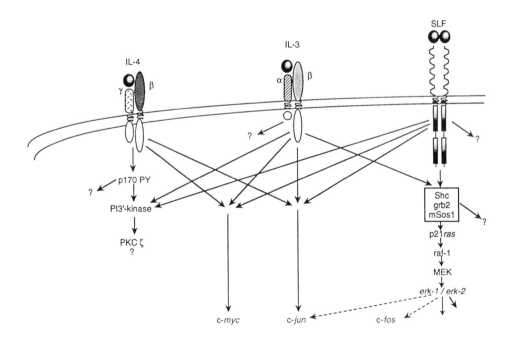

SUMMARY

The action on mast cells of SLF, via a tyrosine kinase receptor and IL-3 via a receptor belonging to the hemopoietin-receptor family induce a series of tyrosine phosphorylation events, some of which are common, and others specific to IL-3 or SLF. Both IL-3 and SLF induced tyrosine phosphorylation of the MAP-kinases erk-1 and erk-2, and of the adapter protein Shc, thought to be involved in activation of p21^{ras}. Both IL-3 and SLF activated p21ras through a tyrosine-kinase dependent mechanism and both also induced a delayed modification of the guanine-nucleotide exchange factor mSos1. However, contrary to the model developed with EGF and fibroblasts, stimulation of mast cells with IL-3 or SLF failed to induce mass translocation of mSos1 or Shc from the cytoplasm to the cell-membrane, raising the question of whether the modified mSos1 and Shc have functions in the cytoplasm. Strikingly, IL-4, unlike other growth factors, failed to induce tyrosine phosphorylation of Shc, modification of mSos1, or activation of p21ras or MAP-kinases in mast cells. IL-4 also differed in inducing tyrosine phosphorylation of a novel cytoplasmic substrate on p170. Primary cultures of mast cells provide an excellent system for the analysis of the molecular bases of the differences and similarities in the actions of various cytokines on growth and differentiation.

REFERENCES

1. Anderson, D.M., Lyman, S.D., Baird, A., Wignall, J.M., Eisenman, J., Rauch, C., March, C.J., Boswell, H.S., Gimpel, S.D., Cosman, D., and Williams, D.E. (1990): *Cell*, 63:235.

2. Bischoff, S.C., and Dahinden, C.A. (1992): *J. Exp. Med.*, 175:237-244.

3. Boulton, T.G., Nye, S.H., Robbins, D.J., Ip, N.Y., Radziejewska, E., Morgenbesser, S.D., DePinho, R.A., Panayotatos, N., Cobb, M.H., and Yancopoulos, G.D. (1991): *Cell*, 65:663 - 675.

4. Bowtell, D., Fu, P., Simon, M., and Senior, P. (1992): *Proc. Natl. Acad. Sci.*, 89:6511-6515.

5. Brown, M.A., Pierce, J., H., Watson, C.J., Falco, J., Ihle, J.M., and Paul, W.E. (1987): *Cell*, 60:809-818.

6. Buday, L., and Downard, J. (1993): *Cell*, 73:611-620.

7. Clark, S.G., Stern, M.J., and Horvitz, H.R. (1992): *Nature*, 356:340-344.

8. Clark-Lewis, I., Kent, S.B.H. and Schrader, J.W. (1984): *J. Biol. Chem.*, 259:7488-7494.

9. Clark-Lewis, I and Schrader, J.W. (1981): *J. Immunol.*, 127:1941-1947.

10. Cosman, D. (1993): *Cytokine*, 5:95-106.

11. Crapper, R.M., Clark-Lewis, I. and Schrader, J.W. (1984): *Immunology*, 53:33-42.

12. Crapper, R.M., Clark-Lewis, I. and Schrader, J.W. (1985): *Exp. Hematol.*, 13:941-947.

13. Crapper, R.M., Thomas, W.R. and Schrader, J.W. (1984) *J. Immunol.*, 133:2174-2179.

14. Downard, J., Graves, J.D., Warne, P.H., Rayter, S., and Cantrell, D.A. (1990): *Nature*, 346:719-723.

15. Duronio, V., Clark-Lewis, I., Federsppiel, B., Wieler, J.S. and Schrader, J.W. (1992): *J. Biol. Chem.*, 267: 21856-21863.
16. Duronio, V., Clark-Lewis, I. and Schrader, J.W. (1992): *Exp. Hematol.*, 20:505-511.
17. Duronio, V., Federsppiel, B., Wieler, J.S., Clark-Lewis, I., and Schrader, J.W. (1992): *J.Biol. Chem* 267, 21856-21863.
18. Duronio, V., Welham, M., Abraham, S., Dryden, P., and Schrader, J.W. (1992): *Proc. Natl. Acad. Sci. USA*, 89:1587-1591.
19. Egan, S.E., Giddings, B.W., Brooks, M.W., Buday, L., Sizeland, A.M., and Weinberg, R.A. (1993): *Nature*, 363:45-51.
20. Gold, M., Duronio, V., Saxena, S., Schrader, J.W., and Aebersold, R. (1994): *J. Biol. Chem.*, 269:5403-5412.
21. Haak-Frendscho, M., Arai, N., Arai, K., Baeza, M.L., Finn, A., and Kaplan, A.P. (1988): *J. Clin. Invest.*, 82:17.
22. Hamaguchi, Y., Kanakura, Y., Fujita, J., Takeda, S., Nakano, T., Tarui, S., Honjo, T., and Kitamura, Y. (1987): *J. Exp. Med.*, 165:268.
23. Hirai, K., Morita, Y., Misaki, Y., Ohta, K., Takaishi, T., Suzuki, S., Motoyoshi, K., and Miyamoto, T. (1988): *J. Immunol.*, 141:3958.
24. Hültner, J., Druez, C., Moeller, J., Uyttenhove, C., Schmitt, E., Rüde, E., Dörmer, P., and Van Snick, J. (1990): *Eur. J. Immunol.*, 20:1413.
25. Ihle, J.N., Keller, J., Oroszlan, S., Henderson, L., Copeland, T., Fitch, F., Prystowsky, M.B., Goldwasser, E., Schrader, J.W., Palaszynski, E., Dy, M. and Lebel, B. (1983): *J. Immunol.*, 131:282-287.
26. Lamy, F., Wilkin, F., Baptist, M., Posada, J., Roger, P.P., and Dumont, J.E. (1993): *J. Biol. Chem.*, 268:8398-8401.
27. Larner, A., C., David, M., Feldman, G.M., Igarashi, K., Hackett, R.H., Webb, D.S.A., Sweitzer, S.M., Petricoin, E.F., and Finbloom, D.S. (1993): *Science*, 261:1730-1733.
28. Lowenstein, E.J., Daly, R.J., Batzer, A. G., Li,W., Margolis, B., Lammers, R., Ullrich, A., Skolnik, E.Y., Bar-Sagi, D., and Schlessinger, J. (1992): *Cell*, 70:431-442.
29. MacDonald, S.M., Schleimer, R.P., Kagey-Sobotka, A., Gillis, S., and Lichtenstein, L.M. (1989): *J. Immunol.*, 142:3527.
30. Miyajima, A., Kitamura, T., Harada, N., Yokota, T., and Arai, K-I. (1992): *Ann. Rev. Immunol.*, 10:295-331.
31. Morla, A., Schreurs, J., Miyajima, A., and Wang, J.Y.J. (1988): *Mol. Cell. Biol.*, 8:2214.
32. Nocka, K., Buck, J., Levi, E., and Besmer, P. (1990): *EMBO J.*, 9:3287-3294.
33. Okuda, K., Sanghera, J.S., Pelech, S.L., Kankura, Y., Halleck, M., Griffin, J.D., and Druker, B.J. (1992): *Blood*, 79:2880-2887.
34. Olivier, J.P., Raabe, T., Henkemeyer, M., Dickson, B., Mbamalu, G., Margolis, B., Schlessinger, J., Hafen, E., and Pawson, T. (1993): *Cell*, 73:179-191.
35. Pelicci, G., Lanfrancone, L., Grignani, F., McGlade, J., Cavallo, F., Forni, G., Pawson, T., and Pelicci, P.G. (1992): *Cell*, 70:94-104.
36. Razin, E., Leslie, K.B. and Schrader, J.W. (1991): *J. Immunol.*, 146:981-987.
37. Rogge, R.D., Karlovich, C.A., and Banerjee, U. (1991): *Cell*, 64:39-48.

38. Rottapel, R., Reedjik, M., Williams, D.E., Lyman, S.D., Anderson, D.M., Pawson, T., and Bernstein, A. (1991): *Mol. Cell. Biol.*, 11:3043.
39. Rozakis-Adcock, M., Fernley, R., Wade, J., Pawson, T., and Bowtell, D. (1993): *Nature*, 363: 83-85.
40. Satoh, T., Nakafuku, M., Miyajima, A., and Kaziro, Y. (1991): *Proc. Natl. Acad. Sci.*, 88:3314-3318.
41. Schrader, J.W. (1981): *J. Immunol.*, 126:452-458.
42. Schrader, J.W. (1986): *Ann. Rev. Immunol.*, 4:205-230.
43. Schrader, J.W., Clark-Lewis, I., Crapper, R.M., Leslie, K.B., Schrader, S., Varigos, G., and Ziltener, H.J. (1988): In: *Lymphokines Volume 15*, edited by J. W. Schrader, pp.281-311. Academic Press, New York.
44. Schrader, J.W., Clark-Lewis, I., Ziltener, H.J., Hood, L.E., and Kent, S.B.H. (1986): In: Immune Regulation by Characterized Polypeptides, edited by G. Goldstein, J.-F. Bach, and H. Wigzell. pp. 475-484. A.R. Liss, New York.
45. Schrader, J.W., Lewis, S.J., Clark-Lewis, I. and Culvenor, J.G. (1981): *Proc. Soc. Natl. Acad. Sci. USA.*; 78:323-327.
46. Schrader, J.W. and Nossal, G.J.V. (1980): *Immunol. Rev.*, 53:61-85.
47. Simon, M.A., Dodson, G.S., and Rubin, G.M. (1993): *Cell*, 73:169-177.
48. Thomas, G. (1992): *Cell*, 68:3-6.
49. Thompson-Snipes, L.A., Dhar, V., Bond, M.W., Mosmann, T.R., Moore, K.W., and Rennick, D.M. (1991): *J. Exp. Med.*, 173:507-510.
50. Trahey, M.F., and McCormick, F. (1987): *Science*, 238:542-545.
51. Tsai, M., Shih, L., Newlands, G.F.J., Takeishi, T., Langley, K.E., Zsebo, K.M., Miller, H.R.P., Geisller, E.N., and Galli, S.J. (1991): *J. Exp. Med.*, 174:125.
52. Tsuji, K. et al. (1990): *J. Immunol.*, 144:678-684.
53. Wang, L-M., Keegan, A.D., Paul, W.E., Heidaran, M.A., Gutkind, J.S., and Pierce, J.H. (1992): *EMBO J.*, 11:4899-4908.
54. Welham, M.J., Duronio, V., Bowtell, D., and Schrader, J.W. (1994): *J. Biol. Chem.*, In Press.
55. Welham, M.J., Duronio, V., Sanghera, J.S., Pelech, S.L., and Schrader, J.W. (1992): *J.Immunol.*, 149:1683-1693.
56. Welham, M.J., Duronio, V., and Schrader, J.W. (1994): *J. Biol. Chem.*, 269:5865-5873.
57. Welham, M.J. and Schrader, J.W. (1991): *Mol. Cell. Biol.*, 11: 2901-2904.
58. Welham, M.J., and Schrader, J.W. (1992): *J. Immunol.*, 149:2772-2783.
59. White, M.F. (1994): *Curr. Opin. Genet. and Devel.*, 4:47-54.
60. Wershil, B.K., Tsai, M., Geissler, E.N., Zsebo, K.M., and Galli, S.J. (1992): *J. Exp. Med.*, 175:245-255.
61. Williams, D.E., Eisenman, J., Baird, A., Rauch, C., Van Ness, K., March, C.J., Park, L.S., Martin, U., Mochizuki, D.Y., Cosman, D., and Lyman, S.D. (1990): *Cell*, 63:167.
62. Wong, G.H.W., Clark-Lewis, I., Hamilton, J.A. and Schrader, J.W. (1984): *J. Immunol.*, 133:2043-2050.
63. Wong, G.H.W., Clark-Lewis, I., McKimm-Breschkin, J.L. and Schrader, J.W. (1982): *Proc. Soc. Natl. Acad. Sci. U.S.A.*, 79:6989-6993.

Biological and Molecular Aspects of Mast Cell
and Basophil Differentiation and Function,
edited by Y. Kitamura, S. Yamamoto, S.J. Galli, and
M.W. Greaves. Raven Press, Ltd., New York © 1995.

7

Activation of Early Response Genes and Cell Proliferation by Shared Cytokine Receptor Systems of GM-CSF and IL-4

Sumiko Watanabe[1], Akihiko Muto[1], Tohru Itoh[1],
Takashi Yokota[1], Atsushi Miyajima[2] and Ken-ichi Arai[1]*

[1]Department of Molecular and Developmental Biology, Institute of Medical Science,
University of Tokyo, 4-6-1 Shirokanedai, Minato-ku, Tokyo 108, Japan, [2]Department of
Cell Biology, DNAX Research Institute of Molecular and Cellular Biology, 901 California
Avenue, Palo Alto, CA 94304, USA

Cytokines play important roles in promoting proliferation and differentiation of hematopoietic cells [1]. They are produced by various cells such as T cells, macrophages, fibroblasts and endothelial cells. Cytokines produced by macrophages and endothelial cells may be important for the establishment of innate immunity, the non-specific anti-microbial response for self-limiting inflammation. In contrast, cytokines produced by activated T cells are the component of acquired immunity responsible for immune defences with specificity and memory functions. Cytokines were originally assumed to be cell-lineage specific and have been named based on their major target cells. This anticipated that cytokines act in a co-linear manner through a series of cell lineage-specific interactions and no cross-talk exists between cells of different lineages. However, cytokines are generally pleiotropic and many cytokines act on various target cells with numerous biological activities [2]. For example, IL-4 stimulates either proliferation or gene induction of B cells, T cells, mast cells, macrophages and fibroblasts [3]. In addition, many cytokines elicit similar and overlapping activities on the same target cells. These results suggested that cytokine signaling pathways are non-linear and form a network with multiple cross-talks among different cytokines. To date, more than 50 cytokines including interleukins, colony stimulating factors, interferons, chemokines, TGF-β or TNF family and growth factors, have been identified and they are known to form complex cytokine network. The response of target cells to a given cytokine is determined by the expression of the cytokine receptor and/or the nature of the link between the receptor and their signal transduction pathways. In general, a receptor complex is composed of several components such as the ligand binding unit, transducer, adaptor and effector. Pleiotropic nature of cytokine actions strongly suggested that the ligand binding unit of the receptor is not the sole determinant of the cellular response. Accordingly, we anticipated that there would be a cross-talk between cytokine receptors. For example, single receptors may couple to multiple signal transduction systems, *i.e.* with multiple transducers/effectors or with a single transducer which is linked to multiple signal transduction pathways downstream. Likewise, multiple receptors may couple to the same signal transduction pathways via common transducers or effectors. This view has been supported by the discovery of the receptor system whose components are shared among the member of cytokine receptor superfamily. Here we discuss the mechanisms of cytokine receptors, especially human GM-CSF receptor (hGMR) and IL-4 receptor (hIL-4R) as models for shared cytokine receptors.

GM-CSF receptor and cytokine receptor superfamily

The hGMR consists of two distinct subunits α and β. The extracellular domains of both subunits contain common structures of the cytokine receptor superfamily, including four conserved cysteine residues and the WSXWS motif. Cytokine receptors such as IL-2, -3, -4, -5, -6, -7, -9, -11, -12, EPO, G-CSF and Mpl ligand (thrombopoietin, TPO) are classified as a members of cytokine receptor superfamily [4]. In addition to these conserved motif, they have short stretches of similar amino acid sequence termed box1 and box2 in the cytoplasmic region. The α subunit is specific to GMR and binds to GM-CSF with low-affinity, whereas the β subunit shows no detectable affinity to any ligands but does contribute to form a high-affinity receptor with the α subunit. The β subunit of GMR is shared by IL-3R and IL-5R and this is the first example of shared receptor system (Fig. 1) [5, 6, 7]. Receptors for IL-6, oncostatin M, ciliary neurotrophic factor (CNTF),

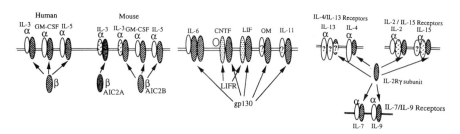

Fig. 1 Schematic illustrations of sharing receptors.

leukemia inhibitory factor (LIF) and IL-11 also share a common subunit, gp130 [8, 9]. More recently, we and other groups showed that IL-2R γ subunit is a component of IL-4R and IL-7R [10, 11, 12, 13]. Pattern of the expression of IL-3R/GMR/IL-5R in various cells are similar but slightly different [4]. IL-3R is expressed mainly on hematopoietic cells whereas GMR is expressed on endothelial cells in addition to hematopoietic cells. IL-5R is expressed mainly on eosinophils and B cells. Because α subunit is unique and has an ability to interact with specific ligand, the response of cells to these cytokines is primarily determined by the expression of the α subunit. IL-3, IL-5 and GM-CSF show overlapping but distinct biological activities. GM-CSF or IL-3, like other growth factors, induces mRNAs of several immediate early response genes (such as c-*fos*, c-*jun* and c-*myc*) and cell proliferation [14]. Pattern of tyrosine phosphorylation of cellular substrates induced by these cytokines are almost the same [15, 16]. These results are consistent with the fact that receptors of these cytokines share a common β subunit. Therefore, we first analysed the role of the β subunit in signal transduction.

Two Distinct signaling pathways of GMR β subunit

We have shown that both the α and the β subunits are essential and sufficient to reconstitute a high-affinity and functional hGMR in mouse cell lines such as pro-B cell (BA/F3), T-cell (CTLL2) and fibroblast (NIH3T3) [17]. We first constructed several cytoplasmic deletion mutants of common β subunit to delineate the receptor domain required for c-*fos*, c-*jun*, c-*myc* mRNA induction and proliferation [16,18]. Our results indicated that two distinct regions in the cytoplasmic domain of the β subunit are required for signaling. One is the membrane proximal region (amino acid positions 455-517) required for activation of c-*myc* gene and cell proliferation (Fig. 2A). Both activities were completely suppressed by tyrosine kinase inhibitor, herbimycin A or genistein in BA/F3 cells. The other region located near the carboxyl terminal side (amino acid positions 544-763) is required for activation of c-*fos* and c-*jun* genes (Fig. 2B). In contrast to c-*myc* mRNA induction and cell proliferation, activation of c-*fos* and c-*jun* genes was only partially inhibited or was even augmented by these inhibitors. More detailed mutation analyses showed that the region between amino acid positions 544 to 589 is essential to activate c-*fos* and c-*jun* genes (Ito et al. unpublished data). In addition, the β mutant carrying an internal deletion within membrane proximal region (amino acid positions 455-517) failed to induce c-*fos*-luciferase activity in both BA/F3 and NIH3T3 cells, suggesting that the region covering positions 544 to 589 is essential but is not sufficient to induce c-*fos* mRNA. Signal transducing molecules such as Ras, Raf and MAP kinase are required for c-*fos* mRNA induction.

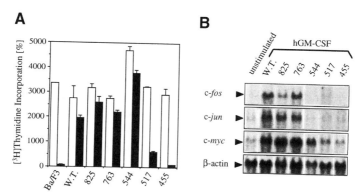

Fig. 2 Requirement of discrete domains of hGMR β subunit to activate proliferation and immediate early genes

Incorporation of [³H]thymidine (A) or induction of mRNAs of c-*fos*, c-*jun* and c-*myc* (B) by hGM-CSF in BA/F3 cells expressing wild type hGMR α subunit and various deletion mutants of β subunits. A; open bar indicated values of cells stimulated by mIL-3 and closed bar indicates those of cells stimulated by hGM-CSF.

Activation of these molecules by various growth factor receptors carrying tyrosine kinase activity have been extensively studied in fibroblasts [19, 20]. They are also involved in the GM-CSF/IL-3 signaling pathway for induction of c-*fos* mRNA in hematopoietic cells [19, 21]. In contrast, little is known about signals leading to cell proliferation and activation of c-*myc* gene, in part because of a paucity of an appropriate assay system.

Signals for c-*myc* promoter activation and proliferation

To elucidate mechanism of c-*myc* gene activation by IL-3/GM-CSF, we performed transient transfection analysis of the c-*myc* promoter (Watanabe et al. submitted). Promoter activity of the c-*myc* gene is relatively weak and had been difficult to establish transfection assay in response to growth factors. We examined several c-*myc* reporter gene constructions using different transfection protocols. Finally, we could establish transient assay of the c-*myc* promoter responding to IL-3/GM-CSF in hematopoietic cells. We found that the region around P2 promoter initiation site of the c-*myc* gene is sufficient to mediate the response to IL-3/GM-CSF signals. Analysis of GMR β subunit mutants revealed that, membrane proximal region is essential and more distal cytoplasmic region has c-*myc* promoter enhancing activity in a manner similar to endogenous c-*myc* gene. Gel shift assay revealed that IL-3 or GM-CSF induces changes of preformed protein-DNA complex at distal putative E2F binding site of the c-*myc* promoter. It should be noted that E2F is one of the molecules likely to be involved in cell cycle regulation [22]. Cyclin dependent kinases (CDK) are also key molecules regulating cell cycles of eukaryotic cells [23]. It has been reported that IL-3 activates CDK and cyclins in hematopoietic cells [24]. Our preliminaly results indicated that the same region essential for induction of c-*myc* mRNA/cell proliferation is required to activate mRNAs of CDK and cyclins. The roles of c-*myc* and CDK/cyclins in cell proliferation has been implicated, but their exact roles are largely unknown. More detailed analysis of the roles of these molecules in initiating DNA replication is currently underway in our laboratory.

Role of α subunits of GMR/IL-3R/IL-5R

The results obtained by analyses of the β subunit mutants revealed that the β subunit is primarily responsible for signaling. What is the role of the α subunit? Because only the α subunit can bind its cognate ligand, it determines the specificity of the response to each cytokine. Does α subunit contribute to signal transduction? To investigate the functions of the α subunit, we first compared the roles of the α subunits of IL-3R and IL-5R with that of GMR by cotransfecting human cDNAs encoding the α subunit of IL-3R or IL-5R and the common β subunit into BA/F3 or NIH3T3 cells (Fig. 3). We found that the reconstituted hIL-3R, in response to hIL-3, activated c-*fos* promoter and induced DNA synthesis in both types of cells in a manner similar to hGMR. Likewise, hIL-5 activated c-*fos* promoter in transfected NIH3T3 cells expressing hIL-5R. These results indicated that the α subunits of IL-3R and IL-5R have properties similar to that of the GMR α subunit.

To examine the role of the α subunit in signaling, we constructed several cytoplasmic deletion mutants of the α subunit. As shown in Fig. 4, cytoplasmic region of the α subunit is also essential for activation of c-*fos* promoter and cell proliferation.

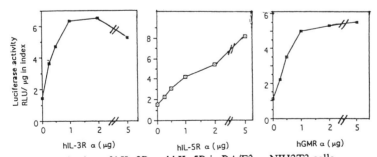

Fig.3 Reconstitution of hIL-3R and hIL-5R in BA/F3 or NIH3T3 cells

cDNA encoding either hIL-3R or hIL-5R α subunit was transfected to BA/F3 or NIH3T3 cells with plasmids encoding β subunit and c-*fos*-luciferase reporter gene.

A   **B**   **C**

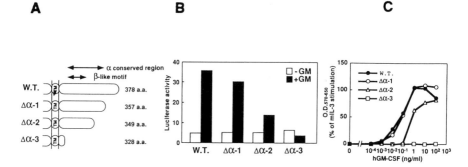

Fig.4 Requirement of hGMR α subunit to activate c-*fos*-luciferase and proliferation

Activation of c-*fos*-luciferase (B) or proliferation (C) by hGMCSF in BA/F3 cells expressing deletion mutants of hGMR α subunit (A) and wild type β subunit. Luciferase activity induced by hGM-CSF was analyzed.

Chimeric receptor of hGMR (α/β, β/α)

We further analyzed the role of the cytoplasmic domain of each subunit by constructing chimeric subunits of hGMR. Both subunits, designated hGMR(α/β) and hGMR(β/α), were generated by replacing the cytoplasmic domains of the α and β subunits of hGMR with those of the β and α subunits, respectively (Fig. 5). hGMRs which bind hGM-CSF with high affinity were reconstituted in BA/F3 and NIH3T3 cells by expressing various combinations of the wild type and chimeric subunits and their potential to transduce signals was analyzed. In transient transfection assays, reconstitution of hGMR(α/β,β/α) and hGMR(α/β,β) resulted in activation of the c-*fos* promoter, similar to the wild type

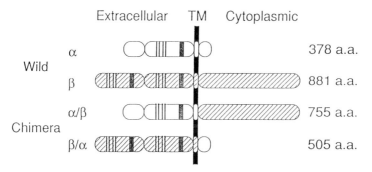

Fig. 5 Schematic illustrations of chimeric receptors of hGMR α and β subunits.

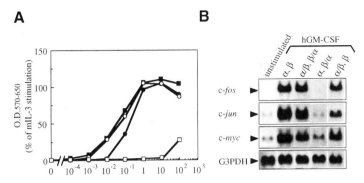

Fig. 6 Activation of immediate early genes and proliferation by chimeric receptor in BA/F3 cells.

Activation of proliferation (MTT assay A) and immediate early genes (Northern blot analysis B) of BA/F3 cells expressing various combination of chimeric receptors. Symbols of A; open circle (wild type receptor α and β), open square (wild α and β/α), closed circle (α/β, and wild β), closed square (α/β and β/α)

hGMR(α,β), in response to hGM-CSF. Likewise, in stable transfectants of BA/F3 cells expressing the same types of reconstituted hGMR but not hGMR($\alpha,\beta/\alpha$), hGM-CSF induced proliferation, activation of immediate early genes and protein tyrosine phosphorylation (Fig. 6). These results showed that to reconstitute a functional hGMR, 1) the original configuration between the extracellular and the cytoplasmic domains of the hGMR(α,β) subunits is not obligatory and 2) the cytoplasmic domain of the β subunit in an oligomeric form is sufficient, without involvement of the cytoplasmic domain of the α subunit.

Role of IL-2R γ subunit in IL-4R system

Sharing of the IL-2R γ subunit by IL-4, IL-7 and IL-9 was discovered as third example of shared receptor system [10, 12]. Initially, we recognized the involvement of the IL-2R γ subunit in IL-4R system by IL-4 dependent T cell growth assay or by c-*fos*-luciferase assay (Fig. 7). hIL-4 stimulates c-*fos*-luciferase activity only weakly in BA/F3 cells expressing hIL-4R. Co-expression of the IL-2R γ subunit significantly augmented c-*fos*-luciferase activity in response to IL-4. Furthermore, IL-2R and IL-15R have been shown to share IL-2R β and γ subunits and IL-4R and IL-13R have been shown to share the IL-4 binding subunit of IL-4R. It is likely that IL-4R and IL-13R share IL-2R γ subunit as well.

These results indicated that IL-2R γ subunit is widely employed by growing numbers of cytokine receptors. However, it should be noted that IL-2R γ system has a unique feature compared to other shared receptor systems such as the β subunit of GMR/IL-3R/IL-5R or gp130. IL-3, GM-CSF and IL-5 have similar, if not identical, biological activities on hematopoietic cells. In contrast, IL-4, IL-2 and IL-7 elicit wide variety of activities even though their receptors share IL-2R γ subunit in common. IL-4 has various activities on T cells, B cells as well as on hematopoietic cells. We previously reported that TUGm2, a monoclonal antibody to the γ subunit of IL-2R, inhibited IL-4 dependent proliferation of CTLL2, a T cell leukemia cell line. Based on this and other observations, we proposed that IL-2R γ subunit is required for the functional IL-4R in T cells. We further analysed the roles of IL-2R γ subunit in IL-4R function in mouse myeloid cell lines and splenic B cells (25). TUGm2 suppressed the IL-4-induced proliferation of myeloid BA/F3 or IC2 cells, as well as of purified splenic B cells. TUGm2 partially suppressed proliferation of B cells induced by combination of IL-4 and anti-immunoglobulin M (IgM) antibody. In contrast, TUGm2 had no effect on proliferation of B cells induced by anti-IgM antibody alone or lipopolysaccharide (LPS). TUGm2 also inhibited IgE production induced by IL-4 of LPS-stimulated B cells. The induction of Class II major histocompatibility complex (MHC) or CD23 by IL-4 was virtually unaffected by TUGm2 antibody. These results indicated that IL-2R γ subunit is differentially involved in various IL-4-dependent reactions.

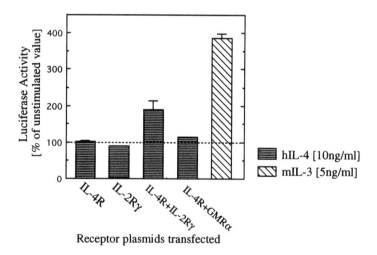

Fig. 7 Activation of c-*fos*-luciferase gene by hIL-4R and hIL-2R γ subunit in BA/F3 cells.

Role of cytokine receptor network in hematopoietic system

Proliferation and differentiation of hematopoietic system are controlled by two types of receptors; *i.e.* the cytokine receptor family and the growth factor receptor family having tyrosine kinase. In contrast, epithelial cells or fibroblasts are regulated mainly by members of the growth factor receptor family whereas lymphocytes are primarily regulated by members of the cytokine receptor family. The growth factor receptor family including c-*kit*, *Flk*2 and c-*fms* may be responsible for constitutive hematopoiesis mediated by cell to cell interaction. The cytokine receptor family constitutes pathways for both inducible and constitutive hematopoiesis and is likely to have evolved along with cellular and humoral immunities. Mast cells are unique in that they are controlled by both types of receptor systems. It is tempting to speculate that constitutive proliferation of mast cells may be achieved through cell-cell interaction mediated by c-*kit* pathway interacting with *Sl* product expressed on fibroblasts. Inducible proliferation of mast cells may be accomplished by cytokines such as IL-3, IL-4, IL-9 and IL-10 transiently produced from activated T cells or mast cells. Generally, signaling pathway within the cell consists of various components such as receptor, adaptor, protein kinase, protein phosphatase and transcription factor. Evidence indicated that signaling molecules at each level are composed of closely related molecules which are the member of multigene family. Therefore, multiple and redundant signal transduction pathways could be generated by combinatory actions of receptors, adaptors, kinases and transcription factors. In this signal transduction network, signaling molecules at each level interact each other by sharing the components. The shared cytokine receptor systems described here is a clear example of such cross-talk in signal network. Further analyses of the structure and function of growing members of the cytokine receptor family and the growth factor receptor family may provide novel insights into the intracellular signal transduction network in hematopoietic cells. Characterization of intracellular signal transduction pathways will also help our understanding of the complex intercellular cytokine network.

References

1. Arai, K., Lee, F., Miyajima, A., Miyatake, S., Arai, N. and Yokota, T. Cytokines: coordinators of immune and inflammatory responses. *Ann. Rev. Biochem.* 1990;59:783-836

2. Watanabe, S., Nakayama, N., Yokota, T., Miyajima, A. and Arai, K. Colony-stimulating factors and cytokine receptor network. *Curr. Opin. Biothechnol.* 1991;2:227-237

3. Paul, W. E. and Ohara, J. B-cell stimulatory factor-1/interleukin 4. *Annu. Rev. Immunol.* 1987;5:429-459

4. Miyajima, A., Kitamura, T., Harada, N., Yokota, T. and Arai, K. Cytokine receptors and signal transduction. *Ann. Rev. Immunol.* 1992;10:295-331

5. Hayashida, K., Kitamura, T., Gorman, D. M., Arai, K., Yokota, T. and Miyajima, A. Molecular cloning of a second subunit of the human GM-CSF receptor: reconstitution of a high affinity GM-CSF receptor. *Proc. Natl. Acad. Sci. USA.* 1990;87:9655-9659

6. Itoh, N., Yonehara, S., Schreurs, J., Gorman, D. M., Maruyama, K., Ishii, A., Yahara, I., Arai, K. and Miyajima, A. Cloning of an interleukin-3 receptor: a member of a distinct receptor gene family. *Science.* 1990;247:324-327

7. Takaki, S., Mita, S., Kitamura, T., Yonehara, S., Yamaguchi, N., Tominaga, A., Miyajima, A. and Takatsu, K. Identification of the second subunit of the murine interleukin-5 receptor: interleukin-3 receptor-like protein, AIC2B is a component of the high-affinity interleukin-5 receptor. *EMBO J.* 1991;10:2833-2838

8. Gearing, D. P., Comeau, M. R., Friend, D. J., Gimpel, S. D., Thut, C. J., McGourty, J., Brasher, K. K., King, J. A., Gillis, S., Mosley, B., Ziegler, S. F. and Cosman, D. The IL-6 signal transducer, gp130: An oncostatin M receptor and affinity converter for the LIF receptor. *Science.* 1992;255:1434-1437

9. Ip, N. Y., Nye, S. H., Boulton, T. G., Davis, S., Taga, T., Li, Y., Birren, S. J., Yasukawa, K., Kishimoto, T., Anderson, D. J., Stahl, N. and Yancopoulos, G. D. CNTF and LIF act on neuronal cells via shared signaling pathways that involve the IL-6 signal transducing receptor component gp130. *Cell.* 1992;69:1121-1132

10. Kondo, M., Takehita, T., Ihii, N., Nakamura, M., Watanabe, S., Arai, K. and Sugamura, K. Sharing of the interleukin-2 (IL-2) receptor γ chain between receptors for IL-2 and IL-4. *Science.* 1993;262:1874-1877

11. Kondo, M., Takeshita, T., Higuchi, M., Nakamura, M., Sudo, T., Nishikawa, S.-I. and Sugamura, K. Functional participation of the IL-2 receptor γ chain in IL-7 receptor complexes. *Science.* 1994;263:1453-1454

12. Russell, S. M., Keegan, A. D., Harada, N., Nakamura, Y., Nuguchi, M., Leland, P., Friedmann, M. C., Miyajima, A., Puri, R. K., Paul, W. E. and Leonard, W. J. Interleukin-2 receptor γ chain: a functional component of the interleukin-4 receptor. *Science.* 1993;262:1880-1883

13. Noguchi, M., Nakamura, Y., Russell, S. M., Ziegler, S. F., Tsang, M., Cao, X. and Leonard, W. J. Interleukin-2 receptor γ chain: A functional component of the interleukin-7 receptor. *Science.* 1993;262:1877-1880

14. Wang, H.-M., Collins, M., Arai, K. and Miyajima, A. EGF induces differentiation of an IL-3-dependent cell line expressing the EGF receptor. *EMBO J.* 1989;8:3677-3684

15. Kanakura, Y., Druker, B., Cannistra, S. A., Furukawa, Y., Torimoto, Y. and Griffin, J. D. Signal transduction of the human granulocyte-macrophage colony-

stimulating factor and interleukin-3 receptors involves tyrosine phosphorylation of a common set of cytoplasmic proteins. *Blood.* 1990;76:706-715

16. Sakamaki, K., Miyajima, I., Kitamura, T. and Miyajima, A. Critical cytoplasmic domains of the common β subunit of the human GM-CSF, IL-3 and IL-5 receptors for growth signal transduction and tyrosine phosphorylation. *EMBO J.* 1992;11:3541-3550

17. Watanabe, S., Muto, A., Mui, A.-F., Miyajima, A. and Arai, K.-i. Reconstituted human granulocyte-macrophage colony-stimulating factor receptor transduces growth-promoting signals in mouse NIH 3T3 cells: Comparison with signalling in BA/F3 pro-B cells. *Mol. Cell. Biol.* 1993;13:1440-1448

18. Watanabe, S., Muto, A., Yokota, T., Miyajima, A. and Arai, K. Differential regulation of early response genes and cell proliferation through the human granulocyte macrophage colony-stimulating factor receptor: Selective activation of the c-fos promoter by genistein. *Mol. Biol. Cell.* 1993;4:983-992

19. Carroll, M. P., Clark-Lewis, I., Rapp, U. R. and May, W. S. Interleukin-3 and granulocyte-macrophage colony-stimulating factor mediate rapid phosphorylation and activation of cytosolic c-raf. *J. Biol. Chem.* 1990;265:19812-19817

20. Welham, M. J., Duronio, V., Sanghera, J. S., Pelech, S. L. and Schrader, J. W. Multiple hemopoietic growth factors stimulate activation of mitogen-activated protein kinase family members. *J. Immunol.* 1992;149:1683-1693

21. Satoh, T., Uehara, Y. and Kaziro, Y. Inhibition of interleukin 3 and granulocyte-macrophage colony-stimulating factor stimulated increase of active ras-GTP by herbimycin A, a specific inhibitor of tyrosine kinase. *J. Biol. Chem.* 1992;267:2537-2541

22. Nevins, J. R. E2F: A link between the Rb tumor suppressor protein and viral oncoproteins. *Science.* 1992;258:424-429

23. Koff, A., Giordano, A., Desai, D., Yamashita, K., Harper, J. W., Elledge, S., Nishimoto, T., Morgan, D. O., Franza, B. R. and Roberts, J. M. Formation and activation of a cyclin E-cdk2 complex during the G1 phase of the human cell cycle. *Science.* 1992;257:1689-1694

24. Ando, D., Ajchenbaum-Cymbalista, F. and Griffin, J. D. Regulation of G1/S transition by cyclins D2 and D3 in hematopoietic cells. *Proc. Natl. Acad. Sci. USA.* 1993;90:9571-9575

25. Watanabe, S., Kondo, M., Takatsu, K., Sugamura, K. and Arai, K. Involvement of the interleukin-2 receptor γ subunit in interleukin-4-dependent activation of mouse hematopoietic cells and splenic B cells. *Eur. J. Immunol.* 1995;in press

Biological and Molecular Aspects of Mast Cell and Basophil Differentiation and Function, edited by Y. Kitamura, S. Yamamoto, S.J. Galli, and M.W. Greaves. Raven Press, Ltd., New York © 1995.

8

Development of Mast Cells and Basophils: Role of c-*kit* Receptor Tyrosine Kinase for Development, Survival and Neoplastic Transformation of Mast Cells

Yukihiko Kitamura, Tohru Tsujimura, Tomoko Jippo, Tsutomu Kasugai, and Yuzuru Kanakura

Departments of Pathology and Internal Medicine II
Osaka University Medical School,
Yamada-oka 2-2, Suita, Osaka, Japan

Fifteen years ago, we found that both W/W^v and Sl/Sl^d mice are profoundly deficient in mast cells, as determined by morphological analyses that detected in the skin of these mutants less than 1% of the number present in the skin of the control normal (+/+) mice. Moreover, we showed that bone marrow transplantation from either +/+ or Sl/Sl^d mutant mice cured the mast cell deficiency of W/W^v mice (12-14). These experiments established that the mast cell deficiency associated with W mutations, like the anemia of these animals, reflected an abnormality intrinsic to the affected lineage, whereas the mast cell deficiency of the Sl mutants, which was not corrected by bone marrow transplantation from +/+ mice, reflected an abnormality in the microenvironments necessary for normal development of mast cells (6, 11).

The *kit* gene was first characterized by Besmer et al (3), as the viral oncogene (v-*kit*) of a feline sarcoma virus. The c-*kit* protein is a member of the type III receptor tyrosine kinae family and exhibits extensive homology with the transmembrane receptors for macrophage colony-stimulating factor (M-CSF), platelet derived growth factor (PDGF), or vascular permeability factor (VPF)/vascular endothelial growth factor (VEGF). These receptor tyrosine kinases have unique features: an extracellular domain made up of five immunoglobulin-like repeats, and a tyrosine kinase which is split into two domains by an insert sequence of variable length. The structure and amino acid sequence of the c-*kit* protein are well preserved among mice, rats and humans (21, 27, 32).

Chabot et al (4) and Geissler et al (7) showed that the c-*kit* receptor tyrosine kinase is encoded by the *W* locus of mice. We demonstrated that the c-*kit* is encoded by the *Ws* locus of rats (27). Shortly after the demonstration of allelism between *W* and c-*kit*, three groups reported simultaneously that the mouse *Sl* locus encodes a ligand for the c-*kit* receptor (9, 30, 33). This ligand has been called mast cell growth factor (30), *kit* ligand (9), and stem cell factor (SCF) (33). We will use SCF hereafter. In the present review, we will described the role of c-*kit* receptor tyrosine kinase for development, survival and neoplastic transformation of mast cells.

DIFFERENT NEEDS FOR SCF STIMULUS BETWEEN MAST CELLS AND BASOPHLLS

All connective tissue-type mast cells (CTMC), mucosal mast cells (MMC) and basophils are offspring of the multipotential hematopoietic stem cell (11, 15). However, developmental processes of mast cells (CTMC and MMC) and basophils are differnt. Basophils complete their differentiation within the bone marrow, but precursors of mast cells leave the bone marrow, invade connective or mucosal tissue, proliferate and differentiate into CTMC or MMC (11). The mechanism regulating development is also different among CTMC, MMC and basophils. We investigated the difference using *Ws/Ws* rats. When *Ws/Ws*, nude-athymic, and +/+ rats were infected with *Nippostrongylus brasiliensis* (NB), the number of basophils increased greater than 50-fold in the peripheral blood of *Ws/Ws* and +/+ rats but did not increase in that of nude rats (10). Blood histamine concentration increased signficantly in *Ws/Ws* and +/+ rats but did not increase in nude rats. Immature basophils increased greater than 10-fold in the bone marrow of *Ws/Ws* and +/+ rats but did not increase in that of nude rats. This result confirms that T cell-derived cytokines are indispensable for the augmented production of basophils and suggested that stimulation via c-*kit* receptor may not be necessary for the augmented production (10).

Next, the role of c-*kit* receptor in the development of MMC and CTMC was investigated by infecting *Ws/Ws* and control +/+ rats with NB, which induces T cell-dependent mast cell proliferation (2). Although mast cells did not develop in the skin of *Ws/Ws* rats, a significant number of mast cells developed in the jejunum after NB infection. These mast cells had the MMC protease phenotype [rat mast cell protease (RMCP) I$^-$/II$^+$] and lacked heparin because they were not stained with berberine sulfate. Globule leukocytes were also developed in the mucosal epithelium of these rats. However, the number of MMC and the serum concentration of RMCP II in NB infected *Ws/Ws* rats were only 13% and 7% of those of NB-infected +/+ rats, respectively (2). A small number of mast cells also developed in the lung, liver, and mesenteric lymph node of *Ws/Ws* rats after NB infection. Although mast cells in these tissues had the MMC phenotype throughout the observation period, the increased msst cells in the lung and liver of +/+ rats acquired a CTMC-like phenotype and were RMCP I$^+$/II$^+$, berberine sulfate$^+$, and formalin resistant. These results indicate that the need for the stimulus through c-*kit* receptor appears to be greater in the development of CTMC in the skin as well as for CTMC-like mast cells in the lung and liver than in the development of MMC.

We investigated the effect of SCF on cultured mast cells (CMCs) derived from *Ws/Ws* rats (24). CMCs developed when bone marrow cells of *Ws/Ws* rats were cultured in the presence of concanavalin A-stimulated spleen cell conditioned medium (ConA-SCM). Although the proliferative response of *Ws/Ws* CMCs to ConA-SCM was comparable to that of control +/+ CMCs, the proliferative response of *Ws/Ws* CMCs to SCF was much lower than that of +/+ CMCs. However, a slight c-*kit* kinase activity was detectable in *Ws/Ws* CMCs, and the proliferation of *Ws/Ws* CMCs was accelerated when SCF was added to ConA-SCM. The phenotype of +/+ and *Ws/Ws* CMCs in various culture conditions was evaluated by immunohistochemistry of RMCPs. Both +/+ and *Ws/Ws* CMCs showed the MMC-like phenotype (RMCP-I$^-$/II$^+$) when they were cultured with ConA-SCM alone. Most +/+ CMCs and about half of *Ws/Ws* CMCs acquired a novel protease (RMCP-I$^+$/II$^+$) phenotype when they were cultured with SCF alone. However, because the number of *Ws/Ws* CMCs dropped to one-tenth in the medium containing SCF alone, the absolute number of *Ws/Ws* CMCs with RMCP-I$^+$/II$^+$ phenotype did not increase significantly. The effect of SCF in inducing the novel phenotype was suppressed when ConA-SCM was added to SCF. In contrast, +/+ and *Ws/Ws* CMCs cocultured with +/+ fibroblasts showed RMCP-I$^+$/II$^+$ phenotype even in the presence of ConA-SCM. Moreover, a fibroblast cell line derived from *Sl/Sl* mouse embryos that did not produce SCF did not support the survival of both +/+ and *Ws/Ws* CMCs but did induce the RMCP-I$^+$/II$^+$ phenotype in about half of +/+ and *Ws/Ws* CMCs when their survival was supported by the addition of ConA-SCM. The normal signal transduction through the c-*kit* receptor did not appear to be prerequisite for the

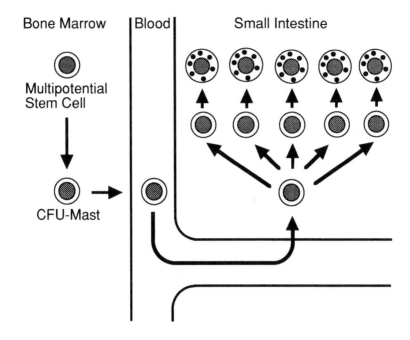

Figure 1. Recruitment of a mast-cell precursor (CFU-Mast) from the peripheral blood into the small intestine and its proliferation after the recruitment.   The recruitment and the following proliferation was induced by the infection of *Nippostrongylus brasiliensis.*

acquisition of the RMCP-I$^+$/II$^+$ phenotype.

We recently studied kinetcis of mast-cell precursors after NB infection. Mast-cell precursors were defined as cells that produced mast-cell colonies (CFUs-Mast) in the methylcellulse culture containing IL-3 and SCF (Kasugai et al, unpublished data). In this culture condition, the number of mast-cell colonies produced by bone marrow cells of +/+ rats was 120 times as great as the number of colonies produced by bone marrow cells of *Ws/Ws* rats. Since the number of CFUs-Mast in tissues of *Ws/Ws* rats was too low to carry out the kinetic study, we only evaluated the concentration of CFUs-Mast in tissues of +/+ rats. The concentration of CFUs-Mast did not change in the bone marrow after NB infection. The concentration of CFUs-Mast in the peripheral blood of +/+ rats dropped to 29% that of pre-infection levels 1 week after NB infection. In contrast, the concentration of CFUs-Mast in the small intestine increased 6-fold. Moreover, proportion of CFUs-Mast in S phase remained in low levels in the marrow and blood, but the proportion significantly increased in the small intestine (Kasugai et al, unpublished data). NB infection appeared to induce the invasion of CFUs-Mast from the perhpheral blood into the small intestine and their proliferation after the invasion (Fig. 1).

DEFICIENT DEVELOPMENT OF CTMC IN THE SKIN OF c-*kit* MUTANTS

Many mutants at the c-*kit* (W) locus have been reported in mice (Fig. 2). The significance of the c-*kit* (W) receptor on development of mast cells is recognizable by countng the number of mast cells in the skin of various mutant mice (8, 13, 28). Especially, point mutations at the the tyrosine kinase domain of the c-*kit* are informative. The numbers of mast cells in the skin of $W^{42}/+$, $W^{Jic}/+$, and $W^v/+$ heterozygous mice are significantly smaller than the value of congenic +/+ mice (28). The mutations belonging to the group showing the severe heterozygous phenotypes are dominant negative mutatious and result from missense point mutations of the tyrosine kinase domain (20, 22, 23, 28). As a result of the point mutation, the c-*kit* protein produced by the W^{42} or W^{Jic} allele completely lacks the c-*kit* tyrosine kinase activity (23, 28). The residual c-*kit* activity was detectable in the c-*kit* proteins produced by the W^v and W^{41} alleles (20, 22). The c-*kit* kinase activity was a little bit impaired as a result of the Wf mutation, but an appreciable c-*kit* kinase activity remained in CMCs derived from Wf/Wf mice (28). The number of mast cells in the skin of homozygotes reflects the magnitude of the remaining c-*kit* kinase activity (28). Since the extracellular domain of c-*kit* proteins produced by the W^{42}, W^{Jic}, W^v, or W^{41} mutant alleles is normally expressed on the surface, none or less functional c-*kit* receptors are formed in $W^{42}/+$, $W^{Jic}/+$, $W^v/+$, and $W^{41}/+$ heterozygous mice. This explains the dominant negative phenotype of these heterozygous mice (Fig. 3).

The W^{37} and W^n mutant alleles are also missense point mutations of the tyrosine kinase domain, but these mutations impaired the surface expression of the c-*kit* protein (20, 28). The c-*kit* protein produced by the mutant W^{37} allele is metabolically unstable, and the surface expressioin of the c-*kit* protein produced by the W^{37} allele is reduced (20). The c-*kit* protein synthesized by W^n/W^n CMCs was truncated almost all cytoplasmic domain and was less glycosylated (16). W^n/W^n CMCs did not express the c-*kit* protein on the surface, and no mast cells were detectable in the skin of W^n/W^n mice. Since the truncated c-*kit* protein produced by the mutant W^n allele was not expressed on the surface, the truncated protein was not involved in the formation of c-*kit* receptor. In other words, the c-*kit* receptors are composed of only normal c-*kit* protein in $W^n/+$ heterozygous mice

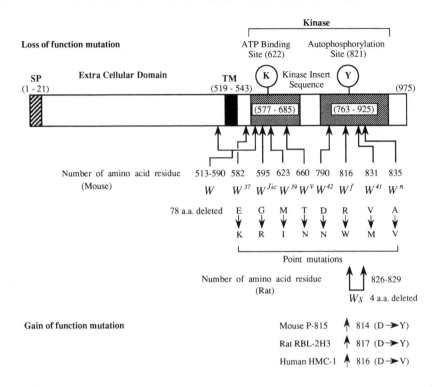

Figure 2. Schematic representation of various loss of function mutations in the mouse and rat c-*kit* protein and gain of function mutations in the mouse, rat, and human c-*kit* protein.   We will describe the significance of the gain of function mutation in the last part of the present review.   The amino acids are numbered from the initiation codon.   The mutations are indicated by a single amino acid code.   Abbreviations: SP, signal peptide; TM, transmembrane domain; aa, amino acids.   From Furitsu et al. (5), Nocka et al. (20), Reith et al. (22), Tan et al. (23), and Tsujimura et al. (26-28).

(Fig. 3). As a result, the number of mast cells in the skin of W^n/+ heterozygous mice did not decrease (28). The number of mast cells in the skin of W^{37}/+ heterozygous mice is an intermediate between W^{Jic}/+ and W^n/+ mice (28).

The Ws mutant allele of rats is a deletion of 12 bases at the kinase domain of

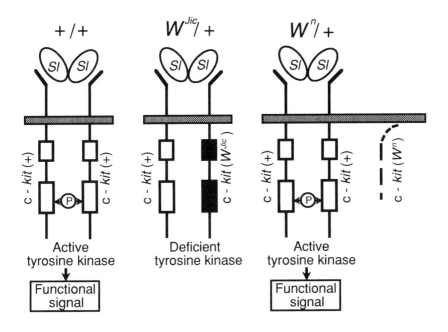

Figure 3. Schematic representation of wild-type *c-kit* receptor structure leading to functional signal transduction (left), dominant-negative signal inhibition caused by the W^{Jic} mutant allele in W^{Jic}/+ heterozygous mice (middle), and functional signal transduction leading to null phenotype in W^n/+ heterozygous mice (right). This schema is drawn after Wagner et al (29).

c-kit (27) (Fig. 2).   Four amino acids encoded by the deleted 12 bases (i.e., Val-Lys-Gly-Asn) are located at two amino acid downstream from the *c-kit* kinase and were conserved not only in mouse and human *c-kit* kinases but also in mouse and human c-*fms* kinases (i.e., receptor of M-CSF).   In spite of the deletion, *c-kit* encoded by the mutant *Ws* allele has an apreciable kinase activity (24), and the extracellular domain of *c-kit* is normally expressed on the surface of CMCs derived from the bone marrow of *Ws/Ws* rats.   With the extracellular domain, *Ws/Ws* CMCs can attach mouse fibroblasts expressing SCF on their surface (1, 24).

The W^v mutation of mice also abolished most but not all of *c-kit* kinase activity as in the case of the *Ws* mutation of rats. The deficiency of *c-kit* kinase activity was comparable between W^v/W^v CMCs and Ws/Ws CMCs. However, abnormalities in development of melanocytes, mast cells, erythrocytes, and germ cells are not comparable between W^v/W^v mice and Ws/Ws rats. (1). W^v/W^v mice frequently have pigmented areas in the auricles, whereas no Ws/Ws rats have ever shown comparable pigmentation. (2). Adult W^v/W^v mice have a considerable number of mast cells in the skin (i.e., 17% that of control +/+ rats), whereas adult Ws/Ws rats have very few mast cells in the skin (i.e., 0.3% that of control +/+ rats) (8, 19). (3). The anemia of adult W^v/W^v mice is severe (the number of erythrocytes is 60% that of control +/+ mice), whereas the anemia of Ws/Ws rats ameliorates with age (the number of erythrocytes of adult Ws/Ws rats was 80% that of control +/+ rats) (18, 24). (4). Most male and female W^v/W^v mice are sterile, and only a few W^v/W^v female mice may be pregnant only once in the young age. On the other hand, most female and male Ws/Ws rats are fertile (19). The signal through the c-*kit* receptor may serve different functions in the two species in regard to the development of the above-mentioned four cell types.

SURVIVAL OF MAST CELLS

The W^{sh} is a mutant at the c-*kit* (W) locus of mice, but no significant abnormalities are found at the coding region of the W^{sh} allele (25). Since CMCs derived from the spleen of W^{sh}/W^{sh} mice did not express messenger (m) RNA of c-*kit*, we studied the interrelation between the number of mast cells and the magnitude of c-*kit* mRNA expression in the skin of W^{sh}/W^{sh} mice of various ages (31). The number of mast cells in the skin of W^{sh}/W^{sh} embryos was approximately 40% that of control +/+ embryos, but the number of mast cells decreased exponentially after birth; the number dropped to 6% and 0.6% that of +/+ mice at days 60 and 150 after birth, respectively. A weak but apparent signal of c-*kit* mRNA was detectable in the skin of W^{sh}/W^{sh} embryos by RNase protection assay but not in the skin of 5-days-old W^{sh}/W^{sh} mice. The number ot c-*kit* protein-containing mast cells was significantly greater in the skin of W^{sh}/W^{sh} embryos than in the skin of 5-days-old W^{sh}/W^{sh} mice. The abolishment of c-*kit* mRNA expression appeared to be specific, because the mRNA expression of mast cell carboxypeptidase A (a mast cell-specific protease) but not of c-*kit* was detectable by in situ hybridization in the skin mast cells of 5-days-old W^{sh}/W^{sh} mice. Taken together, the expression of c-*kit* mRNA was abolished first, then the content of c-*kit* protein dropped to undetectable levels, and then the disappearance of mast cells themselves followed (31). This clearly indicates the essential role of the SCF/c-*kit* receptor system for the survival of mast cells.

No significant abnormalities were detectable in the coding region of the W^{sh} mutant allele. In addition to the age-dependent abolishment of c-*kit* in mast cells, cell type-specific abolishment of c-*kit* mRNA expression was observed in W^{sh}/W^{sh}

mice (25). Although adult *Wsh/Wsh* mice showed a remarkable deplection of mast cells, they were not anemic. Most homozygous or double heterozygous mutant mice at the *W* locus, of which mast-cell depletion was comparabpe to *Wsh/Wsh* mice, are deficient in germ cells. However male and female *Wsh/Wsh* mice have an appreciable numbers of germ cells in their gonads. We investigated the mechanism of specific depletion of mast cells. Despite the lack of c-*kit* mRNA in *Wsh/Wsh* CMCs, the c-*kit* mRNA was normally detecatble in the cerebellum, and weakly detectable in the testis and spleen of *Wsh/Wsh* mice. Development of mast cells, erythrocytes, and germ cells in *Wsh/Wsh* mice appeared to be parallel with the magnitude of the c-*kit* mRNA expression in each cell type (25).

ACTIVATION MUTATION OF *c-kit* AND NEOPLASTIC TRANS-FORMATION OF MAST CELLS

Binding of SCF to c-*kit* receptor activates c-*kit* tyrosine kinase and leads to autophospholylation of c-*kit* kinase on tyrosine and to association of c-*kit* with substrates such as phosphatidylinositol 3-kinase (PI3K) (17). In a human mast cell leukemia cell line HMC-1, the c-*kit* kinase was constitutively phospholylated on tyrosine, activated, and associated with PI3K without the addition of SCF. Furitsu et al (5) found that the c-*kit* gene of HMC-1 cells was composed of a normal, wild-type allele and a mutant allele with point mutations resulting in amino acid substitutions of Gly-560 for Val and Val-816 for Asp. Amino acid sequences in the regions of the two mutations are completely conserved in all of mouse, rat, and human c-*kit* (Fig. 4).

In order to determine the causal role of these mutations in the constitutive activation, murine c-*kit* mutants encoding Gly-559 or Val-814, corresponding to human Gly-560 or Val-816, were constructed and expressed in a human embryonic kidney cell line, 293T cells. In the transfected cells, the c-*kit* kinase (Val-814) was abundantly phospholyated on tyrosine and activated in immune complex kinase reaction in the absence of SCF, whereas tyrosine phospholylation and activation of c-*kit* kinase (Gly-559) of wild-type c-*kit* kinase was modest or little, respectively. The conversion of Asp-816 to Val in human c-*kit* kinase appears to be an activation mutation and responsible for the constitutive activation of c-*kit* kinase in HMC-1 cells (5).

Recently, Tsujimura et al (26) found the corresponding mutation in the P-815 mouse mastocytoma cell line (Asp-814 to Tyr) and the RBL-2H3 rat mast cell leukemia cell line (Asp-817 to Tyr). Both P-815 and RBL-2H3 cells showed constitutive activation of c-*kit* kinase without the addition of SCF. The substitution of the same amino acid has not been found among various mutants of mice, rats, and humans, but was found in the mastocytoma cell lines of all mice, rats, and humans (Fig. 4). There is a possibility that this mutation has induced mast cell

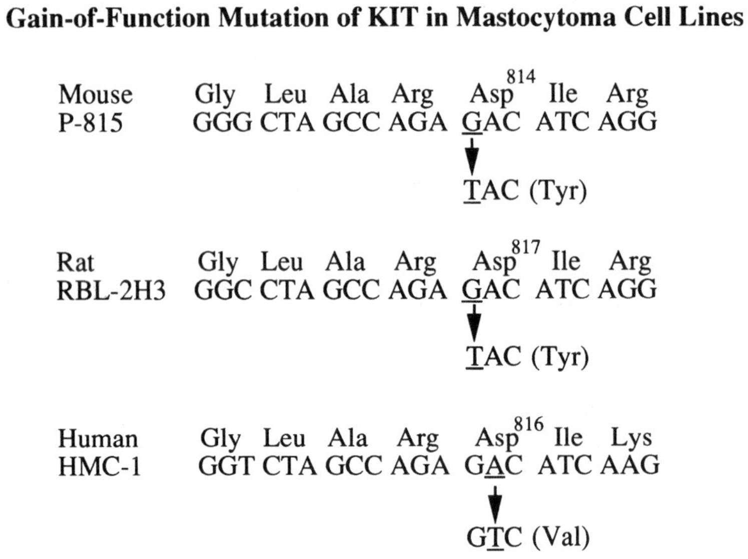

Gain-of-Function Mutation of KIT in Mastocytoma Cell Lines

Mouse   Gly Leu Ala Arg   Asp^{814} Ile Arg
P-815   GGG CTA GCC AGA G̲AC ATC AGG
                                    ↓
                              T̲AC (Tyr)

Rat   Gly Leu Ala Arg   Asp^{817} Ile Arg
RBL-2H3   GGC CTA GCC AGA G̲AC ATC AGG
                                    ↓
                              T̲AC (Tyr)

Human   Gly Leu Ala Arg   Asp^{816} Ile Lys
HMC-1   GGT CTA GCC AGA GA̲C ATC AAG
                                    ↓
                              GT̲C (Val)

Figure 4. The substitution of the same aspartic acid observed in the mouse P-815 mastocytoma cell line and in the rat RBL-2H3 and human HMC-1 mast cell leukemia cell lines.   For the location of the aspartic acid, see Fig. 2.

tumors in the above-mentioned three species. In order to determine whether constitutive activation of   c-*kit* receptor tyrosine kinase had any roles in the factor-independent growth, RBL-2H3 cells were cultured with sense, antisense, or missense oligonucleotides of c-*kit* mRNA, and the proliferation of RBL-2H3 cells was evaluated. The incorporation of sense or missense oligonucleotides of c-*kit* mRNA showed rather a small effect on the proliferation of RBL-2H3 cells, but the incorporation of antisense oligo-nucleotides of c-*kit* mRNA significantly suppressed the proliferastion.   Transgenic mice with the mutant c-*kit* were produced to examine whether the constitutive activation of c-*kit* receptor tyrosine kinase is involved in the *in vivo* oncogenesis. In two of such transgenic mice, leukemia developed. (Tsujimura et al, unpublished data).

REFERENCES

1. Adachi S, Ebi Y, Nishikawa S-I, Hayashi S-I, Yamazaki M, Kasugai T, Yamamura T, Nomura S, Kitamura Y. Necessity of extracellular domain of *W* (c-*kit*) receptors for attachment of murine cultured mast cells to fibroblasts. *Blood* 1992;79:650-6.

2. Arizono N, Kasugai T. Yamada M. Okada M, Morimoto M, Tei H, Newland GFJ, Miller HRP, Kitamura Y. Infection of *Nippostrongylus brasiliensis* induces development of mucosal-type but not connective tissue-type mast cells in genetically mast-cell deficient *Ws/Ws* rats. *Blood* 1993;81:2572-9.

3. Besmer P, Murphy JE, George PC, Qui F, Bergold PJ, Lederman L, Snyder HW, Brodeur D, Zuckerman EE, Hardy WD. A new acute transforming feline retrovirus and relationship of its oncogene v-*kit* with the protein kinase gene falllily. *Nature* 1986;320:415-421.

4. Chabot B, Stephenson DA, Chapman VM, Besmer P, Bernstein A. The proto-oncogene c-*kit* encoding a transmembrane tyrosine kinase receptor maps to the mouse *W* locus. *Nature* 1988;335:88-9.

5. Furitsu T, Tsujimura T, Tono T, Ikeda H, Kitayama H, Koshimizu U, Sugahara H, Butterfield JH, Ashman LK, Kanayama Y, Matsuzawa Y, Kitamura Y, Kanakura Y. Identification of mutations in the coding region of the proto-oncogene c-*kit* in a human mast cell leukemia cell line causing ligand-independent activation of c-*kit* product. *J Clin Invest* 1993;92:1736-44.

6. Galli SJ, Tsai M, Wershil BK. The c-*kit* receptor, stem cell factor, and mast cells: what each is teaching us about the others. *Amer J Pathol* 1993;142:965-74.

7. Geisslerr EN, Ryan MA, Houseman DE. The dominant white-spotting (*W*) locus of the mouse encodes the c-*kit* proto-oncogene. *Cell* 1988;55: 185-92.

8. Go S, Kitamura Y, Nishimune M. Effect of *W* and *Wᵛ* alleles on production of tissue mast cells in mice. *J Hered* 1980;71:41-4.

9. Huang E, Nocka K, Beier DR, Chu TY, Buck J, Lahm HW, Wellner D, Leder P, Besmer P. The hematopoietic growth factor KL is encoded by the *Sl* locus and is the ligand of the c-*kit* receptor, the gene product of the *W* locus. *Cell* 1990;63:225-33.

10. Kasugai T, Okada M, Morimoto M, Arizono N, Maeyama K, Yamada M, Tei H, Dohmae K, Onoue H, Newland GFJ, Watanabe T, Nishimune Y, Miller HRP, Kitamura Y. Infection of *Nippostrongylus brasiliensis* induces normal increase of basophils in mast-cell deficient *Ws/Ws* rats with small deletion at the kinase domain of c-*kit*. *Blood* 1993;81:2521-9.

11. Kitamura Y. Heterogenesity of mast cells and phenotypic change

between subpopulations. *Annu Rev Immunol* 1989;7:59-76.

12. Kitamura Y, Go S. Decreased production of mast cells in *Sl/Sl^d* anemic mice. *Blood* 1979;53:492-7.

13. Kitamura Y, Go S, Hatanaka K. Decrease of mast cells in *W/W^v* mice and their increase by bone marrow transplantation. *Blood* 1978;52:447-52.

14. Kitamura Y, Nakayama H, Fujita J, Mechanism of mast cell deficiency in mutant mice of *W/W^v* and *Sl/Sl^d* genotype. In:Galli SJ, Austin KF. *Mast cell and Basophil Differentiation and Function in Health and Disease.* New York: Raven Press; 1989:15-25.

15. Kitamura Y, Yokoyama M, Matsuda H, Ohno T, Mori KJ. Spleen colony forming cell as common precursor for tissue mast cells and granulocytes. *Nature* 1981;291:159-60.

16. Koshimizu U, Tsujimura T, Isozaki K, Nomura S, Furitsu T, Kanakura Y, Kitamura Y, Nishimune Y. *W^n* mutation of c-*kit* receptor affects its post-translational processing and extracellular expression. *Oncogene* 1994;9:157-62.

17. Lev S, Givol D, Yarden Y. Interkinase domain of kit contains the binding site for phosphatidylinositol 3' kinase. *Proc Natl Acad Sci USA* 1992; 89:678-82.

18. Morimoto M, Kasugai T, Tei H, Jippo-Kanemoto T, Kanakura Y, Kitamura Y. Age-dependent amelioration of hypoplastic anemia in *Ws/Ws* rats with a small deletion at the kinase domain of c-*kit*. *Blood* 1993;82:3315-20.

19. Niwa Y, Kasugai T, Ohno K, Morimoto M, Yamazaki M, Dohmae K, Nishimune Y, Kondo K, Kitamura Y. Anemia and mast cell depletion in mutant rats that are homozygous at "white spotting (*Ws*)" locus. *Blood* 1991;78:1936-41.

20. Nocka K, Tan JC, Chiu E, Chu TY, Ray P, Traktman P, Besmer P. Molecular bases of dominant negative and loss of function mutations at the murine c-*kit*/white spotting locus: *W^{37}*, *W^v*, *W^{41}* and *W*. *EMBO J* 1990;9:1805-13.

21. Qiu F, Ray P, Brown K, Barker PE, Jhanwar S, Ruddle FH, Besmer P. Primary structure of c-*kit*: relationship with the CSF-1/PDGF receptor kinase family-oncogenic activation of v-*kit* involves deletion of extracellular domain and C terminus. *EMBO J* 1988;7:1003-11.

22. Reith AD, Rottapel R, Giddens E, Brady C, Forrester L, Bernstein A. *W* mutant mice with mild or severe developmental defects contain distinct point mutations in the kinase domain of the c-*kit* receptor. *Genes Dev* 1990;4:390-400.

23. Tan JC, Nocka K, Ray P, Traktmall P, Besmer P. The dominant *W^{42}* spotting phenotype results from a missense mutation in the c-*kit* receptor

kinase. *Science* 1990;247:209-12.

24. Tei H, Kasugai T, Tsujimura T, Adachi S, Furitsu T, Tohya K, Kimura M, Zsebo KM, Newlands GFJ, Miller HRP, Kanakura Y, Kitamura Y. Characterization of cultured mast cells derived from *Ws/Ws* mast cell-deficient rats with a small deletion at tyrosine kinase domain of c-*kit*. *Blood* 1994;83:916-25.

25. Tono T, Tsujimura T, Koshimizu U, Kasugai T, Adachi S, Isozaki K, Nishikawa S-I, Morimoto M, Nishimune Y, Nomura S, Kitamura Y. Deficient transcription of c-*kit* gene in cultured mast cells of W*sh*/W*sh* mice that have nearly normal number of erythrocytes and norrnal c-*kit* coding region. *Blood* 1992;80:1448-53.

26. Tsujimura T, Furitsu T, Morimoto M, Isozaki K, Nomura S, Matsuzawa Y, Kitamura Y, Kanakura Y. Ligand-independent activation of c-*kit* receptor tyrosine kinase in a murine mastocytoma cell line P-815 generated by a point mutation. *Blood* 1994;83:2619-26.

27. Tsujimura T, Hirota S, Nomura S, Niwa Y, Yamazaki M, Tono T, Morii E, Kim HM, Kondo K, Nishimune Y, Kitamura Y: Characterization of *Ws* mutant allele of rats: a 12 base deletion in tyrosine kinase domain of c-*kit* gene. *Blood* 1991;78:1942-6.

28. Tsujimura T, Koshimizu U, Katoh H, Isozaki K, Tono T, Adachi S, Kasugai T, Tei H, Nishimune Y, Nomura S, Kitamura Y. Mast cell number of heterozygotes reflects the molecular nature of c-*kit* mutation. *Blood* 1993;81:2530-8.

29. Wagner EF, Alexander WA. Of kit and mouse and man. *Cur Biol* 1991;1:356-8.

30. Williams DE, Eisenman J, Baird A, Rauch C, Ness KV, March CJ, Park LS, Martin U, Mochizuki DY, Boswell HS, Burgess GS, Cosman D, Lyman SD. Identification of ligand for the c-*kit* proto-oncogene. *Cell* 1990; 63:167-74.

31. Yamazaki M, Tsujimura T, Isozaki K, Onoue H, Nomura S, Kitamura Y. c-*kit* gene is expressed by skin mast cells in embryos but not in puppies of W*sh*/W*sh* mice: age-dependent abolishment of c-*kit* gene expression. *Blood* 1994;83:3509-16.

32. Yarden Y, Kwang W-J, Yang-Feng T, Coussens L, Munemitsu S, Dull TJ, Chen E, Sehlessinger J, Francke U, Ullrich A: Human proto-oncogene c-*kit*: a new cell surface receptor tyrosine kinase for an unidentified ligand. *EMBO J* 1987;6:3341-51.

33. Zsebo KM, Wypych J, McNiece IK, Lu HS, Smith KA, Karkare SB, Sachdev RK, Yuschenkoff VN, Birkett NC, Williams LR, Satayagal VN, Tung W, Bosselman RA, Mendiaz EA, Langley KE. Identification, purification, and biological characterization of hematopoietic stem cell factor from buffalo rat liver-conditioned medium. *Cell* 1990;63:195-201.

Biological and Molecular Aspects of Mast Cell and Basophil Differentiation and Function, edited by Y. Kitamura, S. Yamamoto, S.J. Galli, and M.W. Greaves. Raven Press, Ltd., New York © 1995.

9

Mast Cell-Committed Progenitors

Thomas F. Huff, Chris S. Lantz, John J. Ryan and Julie A. Leftwich

Department of Microbiology and Immunology, Medical College of Virginia campus, Virginia Commonwealth University, Richmond, Virginia 23298

Mast cells, like blood cells, are derived from bone marrow progenitors. Unlike blood cells, mast cells do not complete their differentiation in the marrow, but progenitors leave the marrow as ungranulated cells and complete their differentiation in peripheral sites rich in fibroblasts or other cells which produce stem cell factor (SCF). During or after limited clonal expansion, progenitors begin to assemble a beautiful array of metachromatic granules. Developmentally, mast cells exhibit a split identity between blood cells and connective tissue cells. The point at which mast cells diverge from other blood cells may be at the level of the committed progenitor. Committed progenitors for other blood cell lineages are clearly found within the bone marrow. However, it is still unclear whether the majority of mast cell-committed progenitors reside in the bone marrow or in the periphery (Figure 1). In either location, the mast cell-committed progenitor can be defined as **a unipotential ungranulated colony forming unit for mast cells**. However, the difficulty in obtaining a pure population of mast cell-committed progenitors for phenotype studies is different for bone marrow

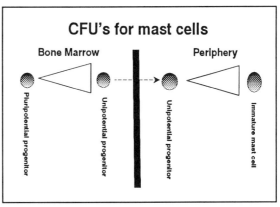

Figure 1. Mast cell-committed progenitors as unipotential ungranulated colony-forming units in bone marrow and periphery.

versus peripheral tissues. In cell suspensions from bone marrow, rare KIT^+ unipotential CFU's must be separated from rare KIT^+ pluripotential CFU's. In cell suspensions from peripheral tissues, rare KIT^+ unipotential ungranulated CFU's must be separated from rare KIT^+ immature mast cells, which also form pure mast cell colonies. These separations are necessary in order to study regulation of individual mast cell-specific genes. Other longstanding questions regarding mast cell biology center on the committed progenitor. Why are there so few granulated mast cells within the bone marrow? Why do mast cell-committed progenitors or immature mast cells which have seeded connective tissue sites develop into clusters which are predictably limited in size (1), given that these sites have a constant supply of stem cell factor? Differentiation of mast cell-committed progenitors may be slightly different in the rodent and human systems. Human mast cells do not respond well through FcγR as mouse mast cells do. Also unlike mouse mast cells, mature human mast cells lack IL-3 receptors (2), perhaps because mice but not humans possess an IL-3-specific β chain in addition to the $β_{common}$ of many hemopoietin receptors (3). Most of the data presented in this review are derived from rodent systems.

COMMITTED PROGENITORS FOR BLOOD CELLS

Committed progenitors have been described for T lymphocytes, megakaryocytes, granulocytes/monocytes, and erythrocytes. Commitment in these lineages is largely defined by the inability of the cell to form colonies of lineages other than the one in question. Sequential cloning in semi-solid medium supplemented with growth factors for multiple lineages is used to establish the unipotentiality of a colony forming unit. Ogawa and his colleagues have studied commitment through the analysis of various colony types produced by the daughter cells of individually micromanipulated hematopoietic progenitors (4). The data suggested that the proliferative ability of unipotent committed progenitors is restricted randomly. Except for mast cells and T cells, committed progenitors continue to differentiate in the hematopoietic microenvironment into mature cells. Mast cells undergo limited clonal expansion and complete their differentiation in the periphery, where their mature phenotype is determined (reviewed in 5-7).

MAST CELL-COMMITTED PROGENITORS IN BONE MARROW AND PERPIHERAL TISSUES

The original studies by Ginsburg and his colleagues (8,9), who showed that fibroblast co-cultures of thymocytes or hyperimmune lymph node cells yielded nearly pure mast cells after several weeks, were in fact studies of mast cell-committed progenitors. Kitamura and his colleagues conclusively established the bone marrow origin of mast cells in a series of *in* vivo experiments (10-12), many of which demonstrated that bone marrow progenitors for mast cells developed into pure mast cell clusters when injected into skin. Precursor frequencies could be determined using these and related *in vitro* assays (13). *In vitro* cloning assays also indicated that colony forming units for both mixed mast cell colonies and pure mast cell colonies are contained with cell suspensions of normal mouse bone marrow (14). Schrader and his colleagues were also able to study the precursor frequency of mast cells using *in vitro* assays of persisting or P cells. Using such assays, it could be established that mast cell precursors were easily detectable in the blood and in the gut mucosa, and that these precursors were committed to the mast cell lineage (15).

Our laboratory has characterized a mast cell-committed progenitor which is present in the mesenteric lymph node of *Nippostrongylus brasiliensis* (*Nb*) - infected mice, but which is difficult to detect similarly in uninfected mice (16,17). These mast cell progenitors intercalate into fibroblast monolayers (18) and form pure mast cell clusters, without exogenous IL-3. They form pure mast cell colonies in methylcellulose cloning supplemented with conditioned medium from either PWM-stimulated spleen cells or fibroblasts (16), as sources of IL-3 and SCF respectively (Figure 2). More recent characterization

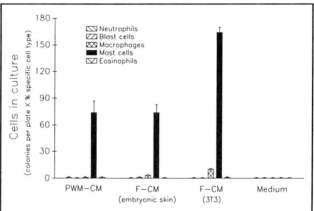

Figure 2. Formation of mast cell colonies from *Nb*-MLN cells taken 14 days after infection. The cell source is virtually uncontaminated with other hematopoietic progenitors. reprinted from Jarboe et al., *J. Immunol.* 142:2405-2517. 1989.

of mast cell-committed progenitors present in Nb-MLN indicated they peaked in appearance 11-17 days after infection and could be isolated by short term culture in Il-3 or based on their density of 1.060-10.70 after Percoll gradient banding. Using an initial magnetic bead depletion to deplete contaminating lymphocytes from *Nb*-MLN, a two color fluorescence sort was performed to gate out any residual lineage marker[+] cells and isolate KIT[+] cells, which nearly all stained with bright rather than dull staining. Of the KIT[+] cells, 50-60% cells exhibited some degree of very light metachromatic granulation. Based on these data and on cloning studies, mast-cell-committed progenitors are 0.05%-0.1% of the 14 day *Nb*-MLN cell suspension.

Mast cells can be easily cloned in methylcellulose from cells washed out from the peritoneal cavity. A number of investigators have described the ability of both ungranulated and granulated cells from the peritoneal cavity to form colonies *in vivo* and *in vitro* (19-22). The ability of mature granulated cells to act as colony forming units is a unique feature of mast cell's plasticity. In these mature cells, the effect on proliferation by signal transduction through FcεRI is unclear (23,24). We have also confirmed by Percoll density gradient fractionation that both ungranulated and granulated cells from the peritoneum can form mast cells colonies. However, the same *Nippostrongylus* infection which causes committed progenitors to appear in the MLN causes them to disappear from the peritoneal cavity (Table I). The results suggest that mast cell-committed progenitors may be effectively rerouted by the *Nb* infection from the peritoneal cavity to the MLN, with likely transit through the gut mucosa.

Table I

Loss of Mast Cell CFU's From Peritoneal Cavity During *Nb* Infection

Cell Source	Day after *Nb* Infection	Mast Cell Colonies		
		3T3 F-CM	rmSCF[169]	Medium
Peritoneum	Day 0	362±35	409±25	0
Peritoneum	Day 5	629±36	ND	0
Peritoneum	Day 8	0	ND	0
Peritoneum	Day 11	0	ND	0
Peritoneum	Day 14	**0**	**0**	0
Peritoneum	Day 17	0	ND	0
MLN	Day 14	139±18	162±34	0

Separation of peritoneal cells from 14 day *Nb*-infected mice gave results which suggested that the low density population was the one which was rerouted, and that in normal peritoneum, these low density mast cell CFU may suppress the colony-forming ability of the high density granulated population. It has been reported previously that in naive peritoneal cells, high density mast-CFU's were capable of suppressing low density mast-CFU's (25). As shown in Table II, unseparated peritoneal cells from *Nb*-infected mice gave no mast cell colonies in response to 3T3 F-CM. The same result was obtained with cells that had a density below 1.082, which includes the 3T3 F-CM-responsive cells found in the naive peritoneal cavity. Unexpectedly, the high density fraction (>1.082), which contained 12.3% mature mast cells and many small blast cells, proved able to form colonies when separated from the low density fraction. The results suggest an active inhibition of mast-CFU's in the peritoneal cavity. In bone marrow, it remains to be established whether a similar inhibition can explain the failure of mast cells to develop there.

Table II
Percoll Density Separation of Peritoneal Mast Cell Progenitors
from *Nb* Infected Mice

Cell Source	Stimulus	Mast Cell Colonies	Percent Mast Cells at Day 0
Unseparated Peritoneum	3T3 F-CM	0	2.2%
	Medium	0	
Frac. 1 <1.082	3T3 F-CM	0	2.0%
	Medium	0	
Frac. 2 >1.082	3T3 F-CM	40 ± 5.0	12.3%
	Medium	0	
Nb-MLN	3T3 F-CM	80 ± 6.0	
	Medium	0	

Fc RECEPTOR EXPRESSION ON EARLIER PROGENITORS OF MAST CELLS

Both pluripotential hematopoietic progenitors and mast cell-committed progenitors/immature mast cells express KIT on their surface, however the committed progenitors and immature mast cells appear to be able to proliferate more near maximally in response to SCF alone (Figures 2 and 3). We were interested in the possibility that, in the periphery, signal transduction induced by immune complexes through γ chain-associated Fc receptors might induce autocrine cytokine loops, particularly IL-3, in mast cell-committed progenitors or immature mast cells. Then, peripheral connective tissue sites , which have high levels of SCF but little or no exogenous IL-3, should be sufficient to induce limited clonal expansion and maturation. Therefore, less mature bone marrow progenitors were tested to determine if they expressed or lacked γ chain-associated Fc receptors on their surface.

Immunomagnetic and fluorescent sorting techniques were used to isolate mouse bone marrow progenitors which express the product of the proto-oncogene c-*kit* but not mature lineage markers expressed by moncytes, granulocytes, B cells, and T cells (Mac-1, Gr-1, B220, CD4 and CD8). These KIT[+] lineage[-] cells were then used in subsequent experiments to evaluate Fc receptor expression during early hematopoiesis. Approximately 98% of these cells have a uniform blast morphology and contain no detectable metachromatically staining granules. When placed into liquid culture, KIT[+] lineage[-] cells were found to be highly enriched for cells

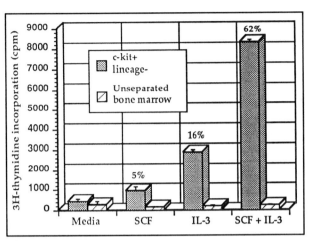

Figure 3. KIT[+] lineage[-] cells were enriched for cells responsive to IL-3 and SCF. KIT[+] lineage[-] and unseparated cells were cultured for 6 days with the indicated growth factors prior to pulsing. Percentage mast cells is indicated above the bars.

responsive to IL-3/SCF as compared with unseparated marrow (Figure 3). KIT[+] lineage[-] cells grown with IL-3 alone or SCF/IL-3 for 7 days contained 16% and 62% granulated mast cells, respectively. In contrast, KIT[+] lineage[-] cells grown with SCF alone contained only 5% metachromatically staining mast cells.

To determine surface expression of FcεRI by KIT[+] lineage[-] cells, we performed 3 color fluorescent analysis of bone marrow cells. To detect FcεRI, cells were sensitized with mouse IgE followed by detection with FITC labeled anti-IgE. Low affinity binding of IgE to FcγRII/III and FcεRII was blocked using antibodies 2.4G2 and B3B4, respectively. Backgating on KIT[+] lineage[-] cells showed these cells do not bind IgE, however high affinity IgE binding was detected on a discrete population of KIT[-] lineage[+] bone marrow cells. Histochemical staining of IgE positive cells showed these cells to be a heterogenous population of various blast cells and polynuclear cells which may represent basophils. These data support our previous experiments showing that incubation of unfractionated murine bone marrow cells with IgE immune complexes increased mast cell colony formation in response to SCF alone (26). The present results present the possibility that the IgE immune complexes might have bound this basophil population to induce production of cytokines which acted on more primitive progenitors to synergize with exogenous SCF.

Since KIT[+] lineage[-] cells differentiate into numerous mast cells when cultured with SCF/IL-3, we examined when during the course of culture FcεRI is expressed. In these experiments, KIT[+] lineage[-] cells were grown with SCF/IL-3 were examined by flow cytometric analysis at day 0-6 for high affinity IgE staining. Cells expressing FcεRI were detected by day 3 of culture and increased through the culture period similar to that seen in unsorted IL-3-dependent bone marrow cultures (27,28). Metachromatic granules were also evident by day 3 of culture with increases roughly correlating with that of IgE receptor expression.

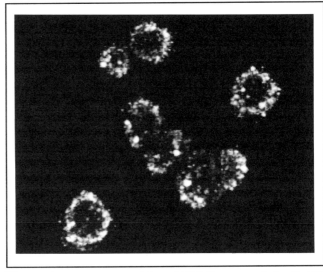

Figure 4. Intracellular staining of KIT[+] lineage[-] cells for FcγRII. Fixed cells were stained with rabbit anti-mouse FcγRII-IC and examined by confocal fluorescent imaging.

FcγRIII, like FcεRI, is associated in the membrane with a β chain and a γ chain dimer, and has been shown to signal mouse mast cells for the induction of cytokine

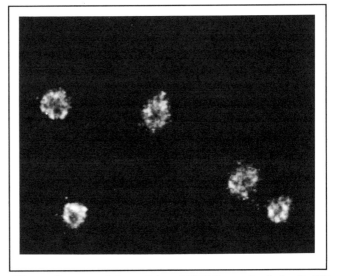

Figure 5. Intracellular staining of KIT[+] lineage[-] cells for FcγRIII using rabbit anti-mouse FcγRIII-IC as above.

biosynthesis (29,30). Because both FcγRIII and FcγRII have been shown to be expressed on mouse mast cells, KIT⁺ lineage⁻ bone marrow cells were first examined for FcγR expression by 3 color fluorescent analysis using FITC labeled 2.4G2. Nearly all KIT⁺ lineage⁻ cells were found to express FcγRII/III. Specific staining was confirmed using an isotyped matched control and also by competitive binding using excess unlabeled 2.4G2. Since 2.4G2 does not discriminate between FcγRII and FcγRIII, we next fluorescently stained KIT⁺ lineage⁻ cells with polyclonal antibodies specific for intracytoplasmic domains of either FcγRII or FcγRIII. Cytocentrifuged cell preparations were fixed and incubated either with rabbit anti-FcγRII-IC or FcγRIII-IC followed by FITC goat anti-rabbit IgG. Confocal fluorescent imaging clearly revealed that FcγRII was expressed at the outer membrane generating a ring-like staining pattern (Figure 4), whereas nuclear/perinuclear staining was seen using an anti-FcγRIII-IC antibody (Figure 5). The lack of surface staining of FcγRIII was confirmed taking Z-axis slices of cells and generating a confocal 3-D reconstruction of the fluorescent staining pattern.

The fact that KIT⁺ lineage⁻ bone marrow cells do not show substantial expression of either FcεRI or FcγRIII argue against a role for these receptors in cytokine biosynthesis in pluripotential progenitors of the mast cell lineage. Recent results in knockout mice also suggest that these receptors may not have an irreplaceable role at any point in mast cell differentiation. Specifically, mice deficient in the α or γ chain of FcεRI do contain mast cells, but they cannot respond to IgE-mediated signalling with mediator release (31,32). Although most mature hematopoietic cells express FcγRII, strong surface expression by early uncommitted bone marrow progenitors was unexpected. Unlike human FcγRII, mouse FcγRII lacks an associated tyrosine activation motif (TAM) present in the cytoplasmic domains of several molecules associated with signaling cytokine production. Since it is unlikely that FcγRII is stimulating cytokine production in these primitive progenitors, the role that might justify such a complete expression has not yet been identified. The failure of FcγRIII to be expressed at the surface may be due to lack of γ chain expression (33). Indeed, using the K1 monoclonal antibody, Ryan and his colleagues have isolated a population of IL-3-responsive metachromatic cells which do not express FcεRI on their surface. The cells contain mRNA for FcεRI α chain but not γ chain (34). To address the question of when during ontogeny or hematopoietic development in the mouse FcεRI α chain and γ chain are expressed, we used a model system based on *in vitro* culture of embryonic stem (ES) cells.

MAST CELLS DERIVED FROM EMBRYONIC STEM CELL CULTURES

One of the difficulties in studying early stem cells from bone marrow is the extreme contamination by late lineage cells. The *in vitro* hematopoiesis observed in ES cell cultures appears to follow a sequential pattern of blood cell differentiation, culminating in the appearance of the mast cell (35). Expression of many gene products associated with hematopoietic cells has already been studied in these developing cultures, but the feature most critical to the question of an early autocrine cytokine loop has not been addressed, that of Fc receptor expression, specifically the α and γ chain of FcεRI and the α chain of FcγRIII. Among the 32 gene products studied (35,36) the only one to be a consensus negative was IL-3. The finding is provocative because it suggests the possibility that IL-3 may not be expressed, at least as an autocrine growth factor, because Fc receptors which are required for its induction, even if they are expressed, may not be used for signalling because no antigen-bridging of passively bound immunoglobulin should have occurred. ES-D3 cells were cultured both in 1000 U/ml recombinant LIF or in co-cultures with STO fibroblasts. mRNA was extracted from 1 million of these cells or from MMC-34 mouse mast cells, STO fibroblasts alone, and peritoneal washout cells which contain mature mast cells. The mRNA was PCR amplified for FcεRI α

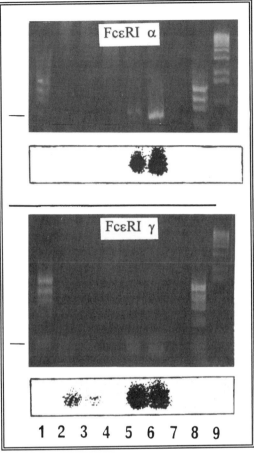

Figure 6. RT-PCR analysis of FcεRI α chain (top panel) and γ chain (bottom panel) mRNA in undifferentiated ES-D3 cells. Southern blots appear below gels. Lanes:1,8, and 9 = MW ladders. 2 = ES-D3 maintained in rLIF. 3 = co-cultures of ES-D3 with STO fibroblasts. 4 = STO fibroblasts alone. 5 = MMC-34 mast cells. 6 = peritoneal washout cells. 7 = no mRNA added.

chain or FcεRI γ chain as shown in Figure 6. Both cultures of undifferentiated ES cells showed a PCR amplification product for FcεRI γ chain which was confirmed by Southern blotting. The Beta scans are shown below the gels. However, the same cells did not apparently contain any mRNA for FcεRI α chain as compared with mature mast cells. The meaning of the early expression of γ chain mRNA is unclear, but the result suggests that the γ chain may have a more fundamental role than just as a signal transducing element in late immune effector cells.

SUMMARY

Mast cell-committed progenitors are unipotential ungranulated colony-forming units for mast cells. They are found both in bone marrow and peripheral tissues such as blood, gut mucosa, mesenteric lymph node, and peritoneal cavity. In marrow they co-exist with KIT^+ pluripotential progenitors, and in the periphery they co-exist with KIT^+ immature mast cells. Normal homing of mast cell-committed progenitors can be disrupted in mice by infection with *Nippostrongylus brasiliensis*, which shunts them from the peritoneal cavity to the gut and MLN. Upon differentiation in the presence of IL-3 and SCF, mast cell-committed progenitors express FcεRI coincidentally with granule assembly. Surface FcγRII is expressed very early during hematopoietic development of mast cells, on KIT^+ lineage⁻ pluripotential progenitors. However, FcγRIII is expressed only within KIT^+ lineage⁻cells, not on the surface. Therefore, pluripotential progenitors for mast cells, which respond poorly to SCF alone, are unlikely produce autocrine loops of cytokines such as IL-3. It remains to be established whether mast cell-committed progenitors or immature mast cells, which respond more near maximally to SCF alone (such as found in the peripheral environment), may produce co-stimulatory autocrine cytokines such as IL-3 as a result of immune complex-mediated signalling through FcεRI or FcγRIII.

ACKNOWLEDGMENTS

We thank Marc Daëron for antibodies to FcγRII and FcγRIII, Jean-Pierre Kinet for clones of the α chain, β chain, and γ chain of FcεRI, Dan Conrad for the B3B4 antibody to block CD23, and Frances White for her assistance with flow cytometry.

REFERENCES

1. Kitamura Y, Matsuda H, Hatanaka K. Clonal nature of mast-cell clusters formed in W/W^v mice after bone marrow transplantation. Nature. 1979;281:154-5.

2. Valent P, Besemer J, Sillaber C, et al. Failure to detect IL-3-binding sites on human mast cells. J Immunol. 1990;145:3432-7.

3. Miyajima A, Mui A, Ogorochi T, Sakamaki K. Receptors for Granulocyte Macrophage Colony Stimulating Factor, Interleukin 3, and Interleukin 5. Blood. 1993;82:1960-74.

4. Suda T, Suda J, Ogawa M. Disparate differentiation in mouse hemopoietic

colonies derived from paired progenitors. Proc Natl Acad Sci. 1984;81:2520-4.

5. Schwartz LB, Huff TF. The Mast Cell. In: Middleton E, Jr., Adkinson NF, Jr., eds.Allergy: Principles and Practice. 4th ed. St. Louis: The C. V. Mosby Company, 1992:

6. Kitamura Y. Heterogeneity of mast cells and phenotypic change between subpopulations. Annu Rev Immunol. 1989;7:59-76.

7. Galli SJ, Zsebo KM, Geissler EN. The kit ligand, stem cell factor. Adv Immunol. 1994;55:1-96.

8. Ginsburg H. The in vitro differentiation and culture of normal mast cells from mouse thymus. Ann N Y Acad Sci. 1963;113:612-20.

9. Ginsburg H. Growth and differentiation of cells of lymphoid origin on embryo cell monolayers. Wistar Inst Symp Monogr. 1965;4:21-49.

10. Kitamura Y, Shimada M, Hatanaka K, Miyano Y. Development of mast cells from grafted bone marrow cells in irradiated mice. Nature. 1977;268:442-3.

11. Kitamura Y, Hatanaka K. Decrease of mast cells in W/W^v mice and their increase by bone marrow transplantation. Blood. 1978;52:447-52.

12. Sonoda T, Kitamura Y, Ohno T. Concentration of mast cell progenitors in bone marrow spleen and blood of mice determined by limiting dilution analysis. J Cell Physiol. 1982;112:136-40.

13. Sonoda T, Kitamura Y, Haku Y, Hara H, Mori KJ. Mast cell precursors in various hematopoietic colonies of mice produced in-vivo and in-vitro. Br J Haematol. 1983;53:611-20.

14. Pharr PN, Suda T, Begmann KL, Avila LA, Ogawa M. Analysis of pure and mixed murine mast cell colonies. J Cell Physiol. 1984;120:1-12.

15. Bieber T, Ring J. In vivo modulation of the high-affinity receptor for IgE (Fc∈RI) on human epidermal Langerhans cells. Int Arch Allergy Immunol. 1992;99:204-7.

16. Jarboe DL, Marshall JS, Randolph TR, Kukolja A, Huff TF. The mast cell-committed progenitor. I. Description of a cell capable of IL-3-independent proliferation and differentiation without contact with fibroblasts. J Immunol. 1989;142:2405-17.

17. Jarboe DL, Huff TF. The mast cell-committed progenitor. II. W/W^v mice do not make mast cell-committed progenitors and S1/S1^d fibroblasts do not support development of normal mast cell-committed progenitors. J Immunol. 1989;142:2418-23.

18. Huff TF, Justus DE. Mast cell differentiation in cultures of T cell-depleted mesenteric lymph node cells from *Nippostrongylus brasiliensis*-infected mice. Int Arch Allergy Appl Immunol. 1988;85:137-44.

19. Waki N, Kitamura Y, Kanakura Y, Asai H, Nakano T. Intraperitoneally injected cultured mast cells suppress recruitment and differentiation of bone marrow-derived mast cell precursors in the peritoneal cavity of *W/W^v* mice. Exp Hematol. 1990;18:243-7.

20. Jozaki K, Kuriu A, Hirota S, et al. Bone marrow-derived cultured mast cells and peritoneal mast cells as targets of a growth activity secreted by BALB/3T3 fibroblasts. Exp Hematol. 1991;19:185-90.

21. Kobayashi T, Nakano T, Nakahata T, et al. Formation of mast cell colonies in methylcellulose by mouse peritoneal cells and differentiation of these cloned cells in both the skin and the gastric mucosa of W/W^v mice: evidence that a common precursor can give rise to both "connective tissue-type" and "mucosal" mast cells. J Immunol. 1986;136:1378-84.

22. Nakahata T, Kobayashi T, Ishiguro A, et al. Extensive proliferation of mature connective-tissue type mast cell in vitro. Nature. 1986;324:65-7.

23. Takagi M, Nakahata T, Koike K, et al. Stimulation of connective tissue-type mast cell proliferation by crosslinking of cell-bound IgE. J Exp Med. 1989;170:233-44.

24. Tsai M, Tam S-Y, Galli SJ. IgE-dependent mast cell activation suppresses the proliferation response to either SCf or IL-3. Eur J Immunol. 1993;23:867-72.

25. Kanakura Y, Kuriu A, Waki N, et al. Changes in numbers and types of mast cell colony-forming cells in the peritoneal cavity of mice after injection of distilled water: evidence that mast cells suppress differentiation of bone marrow-derived precursors. Blood. 1988;71:573-80.

26. Ashman RI, Jarboe DL, Conrad DH, Huff TF. The mast cell-committed progenitor. In vitro generation of committed progenitors from bone marrow. J Immunol. 1991;146:211-6.

27. Thompson HL, Metcalfe DD, Kinet J-P. Early expression of high-affinity receptor for immunoglobulin E (FcεRI) during differentiation of mouse mast cells and human basophils. J Clin Invest. 1990;85:1227-33.

28. Rottem M, Barbieri S, Kinet JP, Metcalfe DD. Kinetics of the appearance of FcεRI-bearing cell in interleukin-3-dependent mouse bone marrow cultures: correlation with histamine content and mast cell maturation.. Blood. 1992;79:972-80.

29. Latour S, Bonnerot C, Fridman WH, Daëron M. Induction of TNFα production by mast cells via Fc gamma receptor. Role of the Fc gammaRIII gamma subunit. J Immunol. 1992.

30. Daëron M, Bonnerot C, Latour S, Fridman WH. Recombinant murine Fc gamma RIII, but not Fc gamma RII, trigger serotonin release in rat basophil leukemia cells. J Immunol. 1992;149:1365-73.

31. Dombrowicz D, Flamard V, Brigman KK, Koller BH, Kinet J-P. Abolition of anaphylaxis by targeted disruption of the high affinity immuoglobulin E receptor α chain gene. Cell. 1993;75:969-76.

32. Takai T, Li M, Sylvestre D, Clynes R, Ravetch J. FcR gamma chain deletion results in pleitrophic effector cell defects. Cell. 1994;76:519-29.

33. Lobell RB, Arm JP, Raizman MB, Austen KF, Katz HR. Intracellular degradation of FcgammaRIII in mouse bone marrow culture-derived progenitor mast cells prevents its surface expression and associated function. J Biol Chem. 1993;268:1207-12.

34. Ryan J, Kinzer C, Paul WE. K-1+, FcεR- long term IL-3-dependent cell lines express FcεRIα and β but not gamma mRNA; evidence for FcεR- mast cells. J Immunol. 1993;150:223A

35. Keller G, Kennedy M, Papayannopoulou T, Wiles MV. Hematopoietic commitment during embryonic stem cell differentiation in culture. Mol Cell Biol. 1993;13:473-86.

36. Schmitt RM, Bruyns E, Snodgrass HR. Hematopoietic development of embryonic stem cells in vitro: Cytokine and receptor gene expression. Genes Dev. 1991;5:728-40.

Biological and Molecular Aspects of Mast Cell
and Basophil Differentiation and Function,
edited by Y. Kitamura, S. Yamamoto, S.J. Galli, and
M.W. Greaves. Raven Press, Ltd., New York © 1995.

10

Molecules involved in the development of human basophils and mast cells

Hermine Agis and Peter Valent

Dept of Internal Medicine I, Division of Hematology
The University of Vienna, Austria

Mast cells and basophils are effector cells of allergic and inflammatory reactions (17,22,38). Mast cells, in addition, are involved in a number of vascular processes. Both cells are myeloid cells representing distinct cell lineages within the hemopoietic system. In common with all leukocytes, they are derived from hemopoietic progenitor cells in response to more or less lineage-specific growth factors. Usually, human basophils complete their differentiation in the bone marrow. In contrast, mast cells usually differentiate in extramedullary organs (17). During the past few years growth factors for human basophils and a growth factor for human mast cells have been identified. This paper provides data and a summary of current knowledge on factors and genes involved in the regulation of growth and differentiation of human mast cells and human basophils.

Progenitor Cells

Solide evidence exists that both mast cells and basophils are derived from multilineage hemopoietic progenitor cells. In particular, in the presence of appropriate growth factors, bone marrow- derived or circulating, colony- forming (progenitor) cells give rise to a mixture of myeloid cells including mast cells, basophils, macrophages, eosinophils or other granulocytes. Multilineage mast cell progenitor cells have first been detected in the murine system (25) and more recently in man (1,23,24). The phenotype and identity of the (uncommitted) myeloid progenitor cell giving rise to human basophils and/or mast cells have also been determined. These progenitor cells express the HPCA-1 (CD34) antigen, but lack IgE- binding sites (1,21,23,24). They express stem cell factor receptor (= c-kit product) as well as receptors for other growth regulators. The immature multilineage precursor cells clearly do not express histamine or tryptase, nor the myeloid differentiation antigens CD11b (C3bi R), CD14, CD15, CD17, or CD35 (CR1) (1). Mast cell- and basophil precursor cells can be detected in human bone marrow, but also in the peripheral blood stream (1,12,17,50). However, little is known about the subsets of precommitted or committed precursor cells which give rise to human basophils or mast cells. A common 'bi-committed' precursor for basophils and mast cells (CFU-ba/MC) has not been characterized so far. In contrast, colony forming cells giving rise to eosinophils and basophils (CFU-eo/ba) are well recognized cells, and frequently can be detected in the peripheral blood stream (12,27). These cells are responsive to interleukin-3 (IL-3), IL-5 and granulocyte macrophage colony- stimulating factor GM-CSF. Mast cell precursor cells as well as mature mast cells typically express large amounts of c-kit (MGF-receptor) and are responsive to the c-kit ligand KL, mast cell growth factor (MGF) (11,45). Studies on purified blood cells suggest that monocytes or blood basophils do not give rise to human mast cells (1).

T-cell dependent differentiation

A number of T-cell derived cytokines are known to regulate growth and function of human basophils. Thus, IL-3, IL-5 and GM-CSF induce or promote in vitro formation of basophils (11,23,35,44,49) and cause basophilia in vivo (18,32). IL-3 is by far the most potent agonist. The same cytokines bind to the surface of mature blood basophils (29,30,46) and promote mediator secretion (20,26,36,46). In contrast, human mast cells are unresponsive to IL-3 and binding sites for IL-3 on mast cells have so far not been detected (47). Interestingly, IL-3, IL-5 and GM-CSF act on semispecific receptors sharing a common ß-chain. Cross competition between IL-3, IL-5 and GM-CSF for binding to basophil surface receptors has been described (29,30). When progenitor cells are exposed to a mixture of IL-3, IL-5 and GM-CSF, no synergistic or additive effects on basophil growth are observed. However, the multifunctional cytokine TGF-ß promotes IL-3 induced as well as GM-CSF induced differentiation of human basophils in vitro (40). A number of other T cell products, including IL-4 and IL-9, did not support development of human basophils or mast cells in vitro. Interestingly, in the murine system, the same cytokines are well known growth factors for mast cells.

Stroma cell- derived growth factors, c-kit ligand

A number of cytokines regulating growth and functions of myeloid cells are produced by stroma cells. Differentiation of human mast cells apparently is a stroma cell- dependent process (15). A mast cell growth factor (MGF) produced by stroma cells (fibroblasts and endothelial cells) has recently been identified (2,14,51). This cytokine, termed mast cell growth factor MGF (also c-kit ligand or stem cell factor) is expressed by stroma cells in either soluble or membrane-bound form (2,14). The molecular forms are generated by tissue- specific splicing. The mature molecule is expressed as an active dimer and acts via the c-kit proto-oncogene product, the cell surface receptor for MGF. Significant amounts of MGF receptors are expressed on myeloid progenitor cells and mast cells, but not on other mature myeloid cells (3,39,48). Recombinant MGF was found to induce differentiation of murine (43) and human mast cells (34,50). In addition, MGF promotes mediator secretion (7,10,41) and is chemotactic for murine mast cells (33). Little is known so far about the factors and processes that regulate expression of MGF in various tissues. Expression of MGF in endothelial cells in vitro is upregulated by thrombin, and less effectively by endogenous pyrogens (4). Another stroma cell- derived regulator of hemopoietic cell differentiation is nerve growth factor (NGF). NGF promotes basophil colony growth and acts synergistically with GM-CSF on basophilopoiesis (31). In addition, NGF promotes mediator secretion in purified human blood basophils (6). It is tempting to speculate that a number of yet undiscovered stroma cell derived regulators of human basophil or mast cell development exist.

Other cytokines

A number of other cytokines have been tested for their ability to induce or promote differentiation of human mast cells or human basophils. The mouse mast cell growth factors IL-4, IL-9 and IL-10 did not support formation of human mast cells in vitro (Table 2). Human basophils express receptors for IL-2, IL-4 and IL-8, but the respective ligands did not induce differentiation of human basophils. The same holds true for MCP-1/MCAF and RANTES, two chemokines that recently have been identified as basophil agonists. The chemokines also failed to induce/promote MGF- dependent, differentiation of mast cells in vitro.

Cellular mediators and surface molecules as differentiation antigens

A number of cell-specific mediators are produced by mast cells and basophils. Mast cells, for example, produce substantial amounts of histamine, tryptase and chymase as well as heparin and. Basophils in contrast, produce histamine, but these cells do not express tryptase, chymase or heparin. Basophil- and mast cell mediators have been used as an objective parameter of differentiation in in-vitro maturation assays as well as in vivo. Thus, IL-3, IL-5 and GM-CSF, an also MGF are potent histamine producing factors. MGF (but not IL-3/IL-5/GM-CSF) induces formation of histamine, tryptase and heparin in human hemopoietic progenitor cells (see Table 1).

In-vitro differentiation of human basophils is associated with expression of almost all basophil antigens including the IgE receptor type I (42) and histamine (49). Cultured human basophils also express myeloid surface molecules such as the complement receptors CD11b and CD35 (Table 1). In contrast, the surface molecule CD17, which is strongly expressed on the surface of mature blood basophils, is expressed only in low quantities on the surface of in vitro differentiated basophils. In-vitro differentiation of human mast cells is associated with formation of tryptase and expression of c-kit. Table 1 provides a summary of mast cell- and basophil differentiation antigens detectable on in-vitro differentiated cells.

Table 1

Induction of basophil- and mast cell differentiation antigens on cultured metachromatic cells (MCS) by IL-3 (day 14) and SCF (day 42) in bone marrow cell cultures.

		expression of antigens on MCS as determined by mAb*							
Factor	day	sIgER	11b	CD15	CD35	CD17	c-kit	trypt.	histamine
IL-3	8	+/-	+	+	nt	-	-	-	+
IL-3	14	+	+	-	+	-/+	-	-	+
IL-3	21	+	+	-	+	+/-	-	-	+
SCF	14	nt	nt	nt	nt	-	nt	+	+
SCF	21	-	-	-	-	-	nt	+	+
SCF	35	-	-	-	-	-	+	+	+
SCF	42	+/-	-	-	-	-	+	+	+

* A combined toluidine blue immunofluorescence staining technique (49) was used to detect cell surface molecules. Histamine and tryptase were detected by radioimmunoassay.

Factors regulating terminal maturation of mast cells; mast cell heterogeneity

Mast cell heterogeneity exists in both the murine and the human system. In the human system, mast cell heterogeneity has been described based on differential expression of proteolytic enzymes (tryptase versus tryptase plus chymase) (37). The human mast cell subtypes can also be distinguished from each other by their response to diverse agonists and expression of surface complement binding sites. The recently discovered mast cell growth factor MGF (kit ligand) induced formation of tryptase in human progenitor cells in long term suspension culture. However, these cells do not express substantial amounts of chymase. Mast cells expressing both chymase and tryptase (MC_{TC} mast cells) were detected in long term culture when stroma cells (3T3 fibroblasts) were used as a source of MGF (15). The identity of the chymase producing factor (probably a stroma cell product) remains unknown. In the murine system, NGF and IL-4 as well as IL-9 and IL-10 were found to regulate differentiation of mast cells and expression of mast cell proteases (19).

Negative regulators of growth and differentiation

Usually, growth and differentiation of hemopoietic cells is controlled by a number of inducing and inhibitory cytokines. In case of basophils and mast cells a number of negative regulators of growth and differentiation have been identified. Thus, interleukin-dependent differentiation of human basophils from their progenitor cells is inhibited by interferon gamma, interferon alpha and tumor necrosis factor alpha (40). TGFß inhibits IL-3 dependent differentiation of human eosinophils but even promotes IL-3 dependent formation of human basophils in vitro (40). MGF- dependent differentiation of human mast cells in long term culture is inhibited by addition of IL-3, IL-4 or other growth factors (50). This might be due to competitive recruitment of non- mast cell lineage cells from a pool of multilineage myeloid / mast cell progenitor cells. The interferons and TNFa also inhibit MGF- dependent formation of human mast cells in vitro (Table 2). Table 2 provides a summary of effects of various cytokines on growth and functions of human mast cells and basophils in vitro.

Table 2

Effects of cytokines on growth and function of human basophils (ba) and mast cells (MC) in vitro

----

Cytokine	Cells	Effects
IL-1	Basophils	Priming for IgE dep. activation. Blood ba and KU-812 cells express IL-1RII. No effects on growth
	Mast cells	No effects observed (HMC-1 cells produce IL-1ß)
IL-2	Basophils	express IL-2R/CD25, no effects on ba observed
	Mast cells	No effects on MC observed so far
IL-3	Basophils	Major regulator of ba, induction of growth and differentiation, promotes survival and mediator secretion as well as chemotaxis and adherence to endothelium. Ba express IL-3R
	Mast cells	IL-3 inhibits MGF dependent growth of MC Mature human MC are unresponsive to IL-3. Human lung MC and HMC-1 cells lack high affinity IL-3R
IL-4	Basophils	No effects on growth or function observed. Ba and KU-812 express IL-4R Ba produce IL-4
	Mast cells	IL-4 inhibits MGF-dependent formation of MC in vitro, IL-4 downregulates c-kit on HMC-1 cells and bm progenitors. HMC-1 cells express IL-4R
IL-5	Basophils	Ba differentiation from circulating progenitor cells. Priming of mature ba, ba express IL-5R
	Mast cells	No effects observed so far
IL-6, IL-7	Basophils	No effects observed so far
	Mast cells	No effects observed so far
IL-8	Basophils	No effects on growth observed. IL-8 induces histamine secretion in IL-3 primed ba. Ba and KU-812 cells express high affinity IL-8R
	Mast cells	No effects observed so far
IL-9,10	Basophils	No effects observed so far
	Mast cells	No effects observed so far
GM-CSF	Basophils	Promotes differentiation in bm and pb ba precursors. Promotes mediator secretion in ba. Ba express low amounts of GM-CSFR. Ba precursors and KU-812 cells express high amounts of GM-CSFR
	Mast cells	Inhibits MGF induced differentiation

G/M-CSF	Basophils	No effects observed so far
	Mast cells	No effects observed so far
MGF/SCF	Basophils	Promotes growth of multilineage precursor cells. Ba precursors and KU-812 cells express c-kit. Mature ba express insignificant amounts of c-kit.
	Mast cells	Major regulator of human mast cells. Induction of MCdifferentiation. Promotes mediator formation and secretion. MC and MC precursors express high levels of c-kit.
NGF	Basophils	Promotes cytokine dependent ba colony formation. Promotes mediator secretion from mature ba. Ba express NGFR
	Mast cells	No effects observed so far
TGFß	Basophils	Promotes cytokine- dependent differentiation of ba. No effects on mediator secretion observed
	Mast cells	No effects observed so far
IGF	Basophils	Promotes mediator secretion.
	Mast cells	No effects observed so far
IFNa/g	Basophils	Inhibit growth of ba. Promotes IgE dependent mediator secretion. Blood ba express IFN R.
	Mast cells	Inhibit MGF dependent differentiation of mast cells
TNFa	Basophils	Inhibits IL-3 dependent formation of basophils
	Mast cells	Inhibits MGF dependent formation of mast cells (human mast cells produce TNFa)
MCP-1	Basophils	Promotes mediator secretion. Induces histamine release in IL-3 primed ba. No effects on growth
	Mast cells	No effects observed so far

Regulation of malignant cells

Only little is known on the control of differentiation and growth of malignant basophils or mast cells. In chronic myeloid leukemia (CML), basophils are derived from the malignant clone (8) and factor (IL-3)- independent differentiation of basophilic cells in vitro has been described (13). The mechanisms of spontaneous basophil differentiation in CML remains unknown. One hypothesis is that factor independent differentiation is associated with (functional) overexpression of IL-3 binding sites. Mast cell leukemia is an extremely rare event. In one case a human mast cell leukemia cell line, HMC-1, was established (9). This cell line exhibits MGF- independent differentiation of mast cells and deregulation of MGF receptor/c-kit (16). A similar, MGF-independent formation of mast cells occurs in a subset of patients suffering from myelodysplastic syndroms or CML blast crisis. In non-malignant forms of (local) mastocytosis associated with inflammation or local thrombus formation overexpression of SCF / kit ligand has been described (5,28).

Concluding remarks

Substantial knowledge on genes, cytokines and mediator molecules involved in growth and differentiation of human mast cells and human basophils has accumulated during the past few years. Studies on these molecules should provide us with key informations on the physiologic and pathophysiologic funtions of both cells in the near future.

References

1.   Agis H, Willheim M, Sperr WR, et al. Monocytes do not make mast cells when cultured in the presence of SCF: characterization of the circulating mast cell progenitor as a c-kit+, CD34+, Ly-, CD14-, CD17-, colony forming cell. J Immunol. 1993;151:4221-7.
2.   Anderson DM, Lyman SD, Baird A, et al. Molecular cloning of mast cell growth factor, a hematopoietin that is active in both membrane bound and soluble forms. Cell 1990;63:235-43.
3.   Ashman LK, Cambareri AC, To LB, Levinski RJ, Juttner CA: Expression of c-kit by normal human bone marrow cells. Blood 1987;78:30-7.
4.   Aye MT, Hashemi S, Leclair B, Zeibdawi A, Trudel E, Halpenny M, Fuller V, Cheng G. Expression of stem cell factor and c-kit mRNA in cultured endothelial   cells, monocytes and human bone marrow stroma cells (CFU-RF). Exp Hematol 1992;20:523-7.
5.   Bankl HC, Sperr WR, Radaszkiewicz Th, Bankl H, Lechner K, Valent P. Increase and   redistribution of mast cells in auricular thrombosis: possible role of c-kit ligand. 1994. submitted.
6.   Bischoff SC, Dahinden CA. Effects of nerve growth factor on the release of inflammatory mediators by mature human basophils. Blood 1992;79:2662-9.
7.   Bischoff SC, Dahinden CA. c-kit ligand: a unique potentiator of mediator release by human lung mast cells. J Exp Med 1992;175:237-44.